Optimize Your Child's Mind, Body and Soul

Nishma Shah

Note to the reader: This book is for informational purposes only. The approaches and suggestions described are meant to supplement and not substitute for professional medical care or treatment. They should not be used to treat serious health conditions with our prior consultation with a qualified healthcare professional.

ISBN-13: 978-0-6923-5251-9 (Custom)

Published in USA

This book is dedicated to:

My dearest children *Kian* and *Sami*, who have been my greatest inspiration behind this book. My loving and supportive husband *David* who has been my rock. My mother, *Niru* who has given me unconditional love and guidance. My late father *Shanti* who had taught me how to cope with whatever obstacles I face in life.

Deepest gratitude to :

My loving friends and family who have supported me in writing this book. To Emma Jamieson, Mita Shah, Jeremy Gilbey and Yubraj Sharma who gave their full heart to us during the first few months of our journey with Kian. To all the special liver kids that have touched my heart. To the medical teams in United Kingdom and United States of America, who have kept my son alive. To all of my teachers who have enriched my life. Finally to everyone who has believed in me and taken the steps to read this book to help improve their own children's mind, body and soul.

"The light inside of me, shines the light inside of you"

CONTENTS

INTRODUCTION

Our first child, Kian, was 4-weeks-old when he was diagnosed with liver disease. I spent days and nights crying, praying and researching all the different outcomes we might be faced with. As time went on, fear crept in especially when we were first told that Kian may not survive.

Thankfully, Kian had a liver transplant when he was 9-months-old, however, we spent two years in and out of hospitals, which was soul breaking. **I figured out early on that I had two choices: give up or fight**. I chose to fight, and I did all I could to learn how to help my child nutritionally, emotionally and spiritually.

Happy and healthy children is what most parents strive for. However, in the 21st century, this does not seem enough. Parents are trying to raise *perfect children.* As such, they want them to be the best at school, best in sports, have a social life, and learn all the life lessons by the time they are ten-years-old.

We are seeing an increase in *stressed* out children, *overweight* due to limited nutritional meals, and a generation that heavily relies on electronic gadgets to get them through the day. I believe there is an alternative in the way we go forward with this, and future generations.

During the last nine years, I have focused on making better choices on what we feed our children. I have introduced them to the idea of inner guidance, and I have used tools to help them stay emotionally strong.

Like most families, our children do have several bad days; however, with the right tools and support, they are guided back to a happy balanced state.

Optimize Your Child's Mind, Body and Soul gives parents the knowledge and tools to break through the 'rat race' of modern parenting. I witness so many adults suffering from various illnesses, and I believe this book will help parents break through the pattern, and help raise healthy well-nourished children not just physically, but mentally and emotionally too. My vision is to see a healthier future for our children.

This book is split into several chapters. It covers:

- Food and your child—you'll learn how different food groups affect your child's body and mind, what to feed your child, and what to avoid. Each section has Q&A, and a summary to help implement changes into your child's life.
- Healthy body—you will learn how the digestive system works, and how it is important to ensure that your child's gut is healthy. I have also gone into detail about the relationship between the gut and brain, as well as the gut's connection with the immune system.
- Soulful diary—by allowing children to express

their feelings and focusing on gratitude, this encourages them to maintain a positive approach to life. There is a diary that your children will write in every morning and evening, which will help them be in tune with their inner self.

- Strike the Yoga Pose—practicing yoga helps maintain a sense of well-being. This chapter explains many yoga poses that your child can practice daily. Yoga gives your children the ability to help enhance their mind, body and soul.
- Meditation—the Dalai Lama once said that, "if every 8 year old in the world is taught meditation, we will eliminate violence from the world within one generation." This chapter explains how to introduce your children to meditation, and it includes several examples you can try with them. Meditation is a gift, and it helps children relax and approach life from a calm place.
- Healthy Meals to excite your taste buds—this section contains nutritional meals broken into breakfast, lunch, dinner and snack ideas. Simple changes in what you feed your children on a daily basis can have a huge positive impact.
- Making the change—this chapter brings it all together, and gives you some practical tips to get started.

PART I
ESSENTIAL COMPONENTS OF A HEALTHY DIET

Our body is complex, and is made up of several different components that all require the correct nutrients to help them function properly. When we are feeding our children, it is essential that these nutrients are present in their meals. Setting a *solid foundation from a young age* will help provide our children the knowledge and understanding that will help them make better food choices throughout their lives.

Your child's body requires a combination of carbohydrates, proteins, fats, water, vitamins and minerals every day. As there are so many different varieties in each food group, it is important that you are selecting the optimal foods for your family.

The wide range of choices available in the supermarket contribute to the parent's confusion with what is classed as '*good food.*' When the large food corporations use clever marketing tactics to help sell their products, this adds further confusion and can make it difficult for families to make the right choices. My favorite caption on some packaged foods is "all natural" especially when, in some cases, it actually contains added preservatives.

In this chapter, I will explain each food group in detail and how it affects your child's body. Once you understand how food affects the body, I am hopeful that it will open your eyes to your child's well-being, and how potentially what they eat can affect their health.

You will become more mindful to look out for

clues to see if a certain food is causing a reaction. With this added knowledge, you will have the necessary tools that will help you make better choices when you are food shopping for your family.

CARBOHYDRATES

The common definition of a carbohydrate is as follows: *"Carbohydrates serve as the primary energy source for working muscles, it helps your brain and nervous system function and it also helps the body use fat more efficiently."* What does this mean? Basically, carbohydrates is our preferred fuel source and children need it for optimal growth and development. While carbohydrates are critical for health, we also need to consider the quality of this carbohydrate that your child is eating. A cookie and quinoa pasta are both classed as a carbohydrate, but we all know which is going to be more nutritious for our children.

There are two types of carbohydrates—complex carbohydrates and simple carbohydrates. The complex carbohydrates such as quinoa pasta, beans and veggies are classed as the "good ones." When your child eats these, they take longer to digest and therefore releases glucose *slowly* into the blood stream. Simple carbohydrates, on the other hand, such as white sugar, white rice, white bread, and all the sugary foods/drinks release glucose *quickly* into the blood stream. These simple carbohydrates causes the body to work harder to eliminate the fast-producing glucose before it can cause trouble.

As an example of how simple carbohydrates affect your body, remember the last time you were at a children's party. **When your child goes hyper after eating party food, you know why!** The glucose from eating the simple carbohydrates is released into the blood stream quickly.

Let's go a bit deeper in the way the body handles this *glucose.* When the glucose enters the blood stream, it sends a signal to your pancreas to release a hormone called *insulin.* Insulin acts like a key and allows the glucose to enter the cells; here, the glucose is used as fuel. It also helps the brain and nervous system function. We need this fuel to help us grow, and also help us get through our daily activities.

When your child's diet is made up of excessive simple carbohydrates such as *white toast, cereals, white bread sandwiches, cookies, chips* or even *soda*, then a lot of glucose enters the blood stream very quickly.

The pancreas works hard to release more insulin that will help transport the glucose to the cells. In some cases, the cells already have enough glucose and they will not let any more in. *So, what happens to this extra glucose?*

This extra glucose is converted to glycogen, and stored in your liver and muscles. The liver controls the blood sugar levels in the body. If the cells use up their glucose (in the form of energy) and blood sugar starts to drop, a signal is sent to the liver to release the stored glycogen. This glycogen will be converted back to glucose and transported to the cells so it can be used to stabilize the blood sugar, and also be used as fuel for further activities.

Just like the cells, you can only store a certain amount of glucose in the form of glycogen in the liver and muscles. *What happens to the rest?* Any excess glucose that is not used up as energy or stored in the liver will be converted to fat.

When we look at the typical American diet consisting of an overdose of simple carbohydrates, an overflowing amount of glucose will be produced. Once the cells are filled with this glucose for energy and the liver/muscles reach full capacity (for quick conversion of glycogen into glucose for energy) then the excess glucose will add to the fat cells. Repeating this eating behavior will cause the fat cells to get bigger and bigger. I believe this is the main cause of why we have so many overweight children in the United States today.

Another scenario; **After a party, do you notice that your child has a sudden high, then low, and then it's tantrum time?** The sudden rise in glucose after consuming a lot of simple carbohydrates in the form of sweets can cause the pancreas to suddenly release more insulin to deal with this excess glucose. This extra insulin could potentially escort too much glucose out of the blood stream, and consequently lead to a fall in blood glucose and your child could be feeling lethargic, tired and grumpy. This process is normally called a *"sugar crash"*.

The way this sugar is handled in your child's body could be the cause of the child's change in behavior.

This *vicious cycle* is what most parents complain about. Tantrums, mood swings, and even screaming can all be caused by this "*sugar crash*". If this eating habit becomes the norm and it is not dealt with, then this up and down reaction of blood sugar can lead to much more serious illnesses.

Assume that the constant consumption of simple carbohydrates become what your child is used to. In time, your child may become insulin resistant. *What does this mean?* If your body has too much glucose, the pancreas will need to produce more insulin to cope with this excess glucose.

With a diet high in simple carbohydrates, the pancreas is continuously producing insulin to cope with the overflowing glucose. One day, the pancreas will not be able to keep up and your cells will eventually become resistant to the insulin.

Your body will have trouble regulating blood sugar, indirectly causing excess glucose and insulin to wander around the body. The excess glucose and insulin is the cause of many diseases including obesity and diabetes.

I am sorry for the doom and gloom, but it is very important to be mindful of what your children are eating. A chocolate chip cookie once in a while is not going to cause too many problems, but when the chocolate chip cookie becomes the norm, that is when we need to be concerned.

How to help balance blood sugar

- Go for foods that release sugar, slowing the complex carbohydrates, for example *oats, whole wheat pasta, brown rice, rye, quinoa, green vegetables.*

- Eat *three main meals* with *two snacks* in-between during the day. This will help prevent sudden highs and lows in the blood sugar. Some children miss eating breakfast, and then have a packaged snack for morning break. This will not only limit the child's nutrient intake, but it will also cause the child to experience tiredness, fatigue as their blood sugar is low. The processed snack (simple carbohydrate) will cause a sudden rise in the blood sugar, and this could potentially cause the child to become hyper.

- Combine carbohydrates with protein. By adding protein, it helps slow down the absorption of the sugars found in carbohydrates. We will have a few ideas in the meals section, but a popular snack in our house is apples with almond butter and veggie sticks with humus.

It is very important to choose the right type of carbohydrates. Selecting complex carbohydrates over simple carbohydrates will help your child maintain a balanced blood sugar level during the day without any sudden highs and lows.

Children need a lot of fuel as they are normally more active when younger. Therefore, choosing the right foods that produce this fuel is very important. Slow releasing foods are far better than your child experiencing a sudden gush of glucose in the system. This is where complex carbohydrates outweigh the simple ones.

Changes in your child's eating habits will be hard. Each individual child will react different to this change. I would keep at it, as the benefits strongly outweigh the consequences of future childhood illnesses.

There is nothing wrong with having a treat once in a while. We personally allow our kids to have a small treat a couple of times per week. What is important is that the "treat" does not become the basis of their diet. **Be wise with your choices.**

Sugar

In the 1800's, the average person would have had about 10 pounds of sugar per year, whereas the average American today eats around 150-180 pounds of sugar per year.[1-2] *I believe this increase in sugar has had a negative impact on the nation's health.*

Sugar is made up of 50% glucose and 50% fructose. The glucose part affects the body in the same way that carbohydrates will (as discussed above). However, this glucose produced will cause a sudden rise in blood glucose, which will put pressure on the pancreas to release insulin quickly to transport this glucose out of the blood stream and into cells, liver, brain, fat cells. As discussed before, the more sugar you consume the more that will be converted to fat.

The other element of sugar is fructose, which the body handles differently from glucose. When fructose hits the body, it doesn't send a signal to the pancreas to release insulin, instead the fructose goes straight to the liver where it is known to potently stimulate lipogenesis (the production of fats).

When the fructose hits the liver, the liver is consumed with 100% of the burden to break down this fructose. The fructose is converted to fat and it starts to build up on the liver and other tissues as body fat; typically the abdominal area.[3] If you continue to eat foods high in fructose, especially the worse kind of all—high fructose corn syrup

(HFCS), then fructose might promote non-alcoholic fatty liver disease.[4-5] This condition was rarely seen before the 1980's, and I believe it is not just a coincidence as HFCS was introduced in the United States in 1975.

At nine months old, my son had a liver transplant due to a birth defect. I have watched him experience pain by not having a liver that functions properly. One thing most people are unaware of is that sometimes you will not have any warning signs that there is a problem with the liver. The liver can quite successfully function even if it is 60% damaged; the only signs that a person may experience is fatigue or vague abdominal discomfort.

What is high fructose corn syrup?

High fructose corn syrup (HFCS) was invented in Japan in 1966, and introduced to the American market in 1975. As HFCS was cheaper and sweeter than table sugar, manufactures began to make the shift from using less sugar and more HFCS.

When a manufacturer uses HFCS, it is named as HFCS-45, HFCS-55, HFCS-90. The number is the percentage amount of fructose contained in that version. For example, HFCS-90 has 90% fructose and 10% glucose. Ninety percent (90%) of fructose goes straight to the liver where it is converted to fat. This will sit on the liver or fat cells in the body.

The problem we are facing is that HFCS is hidden in so many foods that most families are unaware that it is present in the first place. For example, it can be found in tomato sauces, biscuits, cereals, drinks, and even cough syrups...the list goes on. It can be very easy to incorporate a lot of HFCS on a daily basis just by eating some common foods.

In 2010, a research study found that children who had excess fructose intake caused visceral fat cells to mature.[6] This was the starting point of gaining a big belly, and is a potential future risk for heart disease and diabetes.

What about Fruit?

Fruit is the old fashioned way of receiving our fructose. The difference between this source of fructose and HFCS is that the fruit and vegetables are balanced by the fiber, vitamins, enzymes and other properties which actually slow down the sugar digestion and help the body deal with it more easily.

Is sugar addictive?

Sugar is linked to pleasure whereby when we eat sugar, it stimulates the brain's reward center through the neurotransmitter dopamine. There are dopamine receptors all over the brain, and this is where we get the feeling of pleasure. If you want to feel good, you will crave what makes you feel good. So, for a child, they may eat a sweet treat and the process of dopamine is released, and they go into a happy state. They want to keep feeling this way so they may grab another treat, or go into a tantrum if they can't have another sweet.

After some time we become addicted to sugar, this will affect the number of active dopamine receptors left in the brain.[7] As these receptors decrease, people are more likely to crave things like sugar just to boost their dopamine levels i.e., Feel good factor. As a disadvantage, when these receptors are limited, your child will need to consume more sugar than previously to keep the receptors active.

When you watch a child eat a whole tub of ice-cream, the pleasure is instantaneous and they feel happy. As they keep eating it, the dopamine will peak. Some children learn to stop and move on, but others will keep eating the entire tub. Watch them after they have finished. Do they look happy, or do they look worn out and sad? This could be a sign that the child is addicted to sugar. And, they may find it hard to stop eating sugar.

How to reduce the amount of sugar your child is eating

From the information above, you have learned how eating the right carbohydrates and eating regularly helps to limit sudden ups and downs to your child's blood sugar. You also learned about the effect that sugar (in all forms) has on the body, and how excessive consumption can be detrimental to your child's health.

So, how can we wean them off it?

- First, focus on blood sugar balance. Be mindful that your child will need breakfast, lunch, dinner and a couple of snacks in between. If you ensure that you cover these meals with wholesome foods, then your child's blood sugar should remain stable and they are less likely to crave something sweet.
- Then, look at each meal and snack, and see where sugar is coming from. *Remember those hidden sources.* By recognizing where the sugar is coming from, you can actually add up to see how much your child is eating. You may be shocked to discover the answer.
- Once you have highlighted the foods, then make simple gradual changes. For example, switch out that biscuit for a lower sugar alternative. However, be aware of added sweeteners as this will have a worse effect on the body. Even if you swap out a biscuit that has HFCS as an ingredient to one that only has

2gm of sugar, then you are still making a positive change. After your child adjusts to this change, then you can go for a healthier option. Sometimes, if we go from bad to good in one swoop, your child may resist the sudden change.

- Be the change. If you eat less sugary foods and eat more nourishing foods, your children will see this and it may be easier to make the change. Also, if it is not in your home, then they are not likely to eat it. '*Out of sight, out of mind.*'

It can be very difficult and time-consuming to figure out what is healthy and what is not. Large corporations use clever marketing tactics to fool most people. With the information you have learned, you can make a positive change for your family and yourself. By implementing the changes now, you can have a positive impact on your child's future well-being. Giving them the tools and knowledge at a young age is the best gift you can give your children. This may give them the leverage they need to protect themselves in the future from the many illnesses that adults are faced with today.

Carbohydrate questions & answers

My children have Froot Loops for breakfast. I am now worried about how this will affect them?

Advertising may confuse you with terms like 'natural ingredients', 'whole grain' etc. and you may think they are good for your child. However, like most cereals, Froot Loops are full of sugar. Roughly, each serving has 12g of sugar which is equal to three sugar cubes. With Froot Loops, there is also food colorings, food additives and hydrogenated oils. All of these additives will affect the brain. I advise you to wean your children off of Froot Loops and choose a cereal without any added colors/chemicals. Once they get used to that cereal, keep choosing one that has less and less sugar. Ideally, the cereal should only have whole grains and a little sugar. It may take a few weeks but small gradual steps each week will help.

I've heard other forms of sugar (raw sugar, honey, maple syrup) are better than processed sugar (like white sugar) and pancake syrups, is this true?

All sugars are bad for your body. They cause the blood sugar to rise quickly and a surge of glucose hits your brain, liver and cells. The difference in 'sugar' is the amount of fructose that it contains. Fructose goes straight to the liver, and this can be an issue if you are consuming a lot of it. With everything, moderation is key. If your child is having pancakes every day with loads of syrup, then that is going to cause damage; however, if they have pancakes occasionally, then it should be fine (unless they have an underlying health issue).

My child eats cereal for breakfast, packaged snacks, white bread sandwiches and pizza for dinner. What advice can you give me on making a change to reduce the simple carbohydrates in his diet?

I am pleased you noticed that your child is eating too many simple carbohydrates. I would change one thing at a time, as going from the current diet to eating all vegetables will not work. First thing to look at is the ingredients. Make a simple swap from foods with a lot of additives to foods that may have a couple. Second, I would choose half white/half whole-wheat bread. For the pizza, choose a brand that also has less additives and chemicals. A great tip is to read the list, and if there is anything you can't pronounce, or if it has more than five ingredients, then it is probably not going to do you any good. There are healthier options out there, you need to investigate these brands in your local supermarkets.

How do I control what my child eats? He will scream and shout if I don't give him a cookie after school.

This is probably linked to his blood sugar levels. If we don't eat regularly, our blood sugar will drop. When it is down for a long time, the first thing we crave is sugar. For your son, you need to check on what he is eating for lunch and if he is eating all of it. Sometimes at school, children get distracted at lunchtime and may not eat all of their lunch.

This will affect their blood sugar. So, when he finishes school, as his blood sugar has dropped, the first thing he wants when he sees you is sugar i.e., the cookie.

What is your opinion on fruit?

Fruit is fructose, and I mentioned earlier how fructose can be damaging to the liver. However, with fruit, the added fibre, vitamins and minerals lessen the burden it has on the liver. As fruit digests very quickly, I would not give it to your child after a meal, as it will start to ferment on top of the main meal. Instead, give fruit as a snack in-between meals.

All the snacks I buy have high fructose corn syrup, what can I do?

Simple answer—change the snacks. There are plenty of snacks out there that do not contain HFCS or any other chemical. You will have to spend some extra time checking the snack sections.

My kids like ice creams, especially on hot days, but I understand they're high in sugar and I don't want to give them ones with artificial sugar, so what's the alternative? What about ice lollies?

With everything, there are so many different varieties available out there. You have some ice creams with 40g of sugar, and others with 6g of sugar. Apart from making ice cream at home, you will never really know what goes into the ice-cream that you purchase at the supermarket or your favorite ice cream shop. In our home, I allow my children to eat ice cream, but I give them small portions, but not every day. As with ice lollies, these are easy to make at home. You get some fresh juice and add some fruit like strawberries or blueberries. Pour them into the mold and freeze... This way, you can control the ingredients.

Carbohydrate Summary:

- *When you are considering carbohydrates, I would choose complex carbohydrates over simple carbohydrates. This will help stabilize your child's blood sugar, reducing their need for the 'quick' sugar fix.*
- *When glucose slowly enters the the blood stream (after eating complex carbohydrates), it will put less pressure on the pancreas to release insulin.*
- *Ensure that your child is eating three main meals with two snacks in-between during the day. This will help prevent sudden highs and lows in the blood sugar.*
- *Watch out for sugar, as it can be hidden in many foods that your child might be eating.*
- *Eliminate High Fructose Corn Syrup, from your child's diet. When consumed in high quantities, it can be detrimental to your child's health.*
- *By making small, gradual changes each week, your child is more likely to agree and accept the changes.*

PROTEIN

Protein provides your child with the necessary amino acids, which are the essential building blocks of life. Amino acids are needed to build and repair muscle, organs, enzymes and neurotransmitters which send messages to and from your brain. It is, therefore, important to provide your children with an **ample** supply of **healthy** protein to help them grow and develop properly.

There are twenty different amino acids you need for good health. Our body can make eleven of these but the remaining nine (which are termed as **essential amino acids**) come from our diet intake.

When considering the protein portion of your meals, it is important to understand the difference between a *'complete' protein and an 'incomplete' protein.*

A "complete" protein will contain all nine of these essential amino acids, whereas "incomplete" proteins will contain slightly less than the nine. Let's go deeper into what this means, and how we can choose the healthiest option for our family.

Meat, *fish*, *poultry*, *eggs*, and *dairy* are examples of traditional "complete" proteins. They contain all of the essential nine amino acids and aide the body to produce the other eleven.

Animal flesh may be a complete protein but it is also full of saturated fat, cholesterol and may be full of hormones and antibiotics depending on the way it was raised and fed. Therefore, it is important to consider the quality of the complete protein that you purchase.

For example, when considering beef, it is important to know *how the cow lived, what it was fed, and how it was cared for.* Was it given daily antibiotics to prevent it from getting sick? Was it given growth hormones to make it fatter? Was it fed grass or other feed which may potentially contain genetically modified organisms, or was it able to walk outside freely? A genetically modified organism (GMO) is any organism whose genetic material has been altered using genetic engineering techniques. While it is difficult to obtain these answers, all of these aspects will affect the quality of the meat, and subsequently the nutrient value as well. **Next time your child is eating a beef burger, consider the questions above and whether you believe there is any hidden nasties that may be present in the meat and consequently transferred to your child after he/she has eaten it.**

I have many people, especially vegetarians, who are concerned about complete protein intake. A large number of people are unaware that many *plant-based foods* have complete proteins also. For example, *quinoa, buckwheat,* and *hempseed* are all good alternative sources of the traditional "meat" based complete proteins.

Now, let's go into "incomplete" proteins. Examples of incomplete protein foods include *grains*, *nuts*, *seeds*, *beans*, *lentils*, *peas*, and even *broccoli*. Unlike complete proteins, the way incomplete proteins work is by combining two protein foods to ensure all of the essential amino acids are being absorbed, for example, combining lentils with rice.

It is, therefore, very important as a vegetarian to ensure that a well-balanced diet consists of a variety of beans, lentils, nuts, seeds and grains. This will help to ensure that the daily protein requirement is met.

Like carbohydrates, it is all about the *choices* you make. If your child is used to eating meat, then be mindful of where this meat comes from. If your child is a vegetarian, then pay extra attention to how you are combining foods to ensure that your child is consuming all of the amino acids needed for healthy growth and development.

An added point is that we also need to be aware of the *quantity* of the protein that our children are eating. I have seen too many children eating excessive amounts of meat. Overdosing on *meat* protein is one reason why children have become so unhealthy. Not only is this meat full of saturated fats and cholesterol, it is also causes inflammation. Therefore, this excessive meat protein in children's modern diet could be adding to the obesity epidemic that our country is faced with today.[1]

I understand that in our busy everyday lives, some families are rushed continuously and take-out food is often an easier option when considering what to feed their children. Also, in some cases, fast food is actually cheaper than purchasing fresh food products at the supermarket. This makes take-out a much more appealing and cheaper choice. This may not be the right choice but if families have no real knowledge about the impact of fast food on their children, then how can they make better choices?

Many families are unaware of the health risks associated with excessive meat consumption. I hate to say this, but a diet made up of fast food is an early death sentence.[2] To keep the price of the meals down, most of the fast food places will not always use the most optimal nutrients.[3]

Making wise choices as a parent can help ensure that your child is fed the best quality protein out there. A question to ask yourself is "**Will this protein nourish or damage my child's health?**"

On the other hand, it is important that your children are consuming enough protein daily. The common characteristic of pot belly with skinny legs and arms is rarely seen in the western world, however, as protein is essential for the neurons in your brain to interact with each other, it is crucial that your child eats enough protein to ensure that the *brain* is fueled to work properly.

I will discuss in detail later about the neurotransmitters in the brain chapter but just as an introduction point, I wanted to talk about the amino acids that are important. The amino acid Tryptophan is needed so the brain can make the calming neurotransmitter serotonin. Serotonin keeps us happy and improves our mood by banishing the blues. Tryptophan is found in many foods including *cottage cheese*, *tofu*, *bananas*, *hazelnuts*, *chocolate*, *avocado* and *broccoli*.

Another amino acid Phenylalanine is needed to make the neurotransmitter dopamine, adrenaline and noradrenaline. These neurotransmitters make us feel good and helps keep us energized and alert. Eggs, dairy, meat, legumes and nuts are high in phenylalanine. *So, there is a link with the foods we eat and the way we feel.*

It is important that our children are getting enough protein in their diet. Like everything else, it's about balance, as too much or too little can both cause problems.

Be mindful of the amount of protein that your child is eating, and be aware of the quality of this protein. If you are a vegetarian, please ensure that you are combining different types of protein to ensure that your child is getting the right amount to produce the essential amino acids.

Protein questions & answers

We are one of those families who feed our children McDonald's once a week. What do you suggest we do to help wean our children off it?

McDonald's, like most fast food places, add various additives that can potentially make your child crave more. If eating McDonald's has become the norm for the weekends, then you will have to make a change to say once every two weeks, and then once a month, and if your children can handle it then only "on special occasions." Remember, you are in control of what your children eat. They may cry and get in a mood, but it's for their best interest. Children are trainable. They will not sulk for too long.

I have heard that fish is a better alternative than beef or chicken. However, I am concerned about which fish is the best?

Oily fish is good for the brain. It has essential fatty acids which is the building blocks of the brain. Salmon, tuna, sardines, and mackerel are all good choices. When choosing fish, aim for wild rather than farmed.

I am confused with the quality of the meat we should aim for? How do I know it is optimal?

Some farmers give their animals daily antibiotics and growth hormones to beef up the meat. These will be present in the meat when you eat it. Some will feed them soy or corn, which is normally GMO. Therefore, in my opinion, it is best to eat grass fed and antibiotic, or growth hormone free meat. Your best option is opting for organic meat, which may be a little more expensive.

As a vegetarian, we have to have more than two varieties of protein daily. Can you explain why?

Each day, it is vital that your body has the right amino acids in order to function properly. The essential amino acids are found whole in meat and in only some vegetarian options. So, it is important to eat 2-3 different varieties of protein per day to ensure that your intake of essential amino acids is optimal. For example, beans, lentils, dairy, nuts, seeds and even green vegetables.

My child eats a meat-based school lunch daily. What can I do to reduce her meat intake?

You can reduce her meat intake to once a day, and then from there you can try 'meatless Monday.' This is a popular theme that a lot of people try every Monday.

My son has been very hyper recently. He doesn't have much sugar so I am wondering if he has enough protein in his diet to produce the neurotransmitters?

Firstly, I would keep a weekly diary of everything that he is eating. Once the week is up, analyze how much protein and sugar he has eaten. One thing to be mindful of is that there is hidden sugar in many meals. With protein, have a look at the sources of protein. The quality of the protein will affect the amount of goodness that will be in the meat or the vegetarian option. Once you have done this, you will be able to see if he is actually is having too much sugar, or if he needs more protein.

Protein Summary

- *Ensure that your child is eating enough protein daily to guarantee that all of the amino acids are being consumed.*
- *Like carbohydrates, you have a choice on which type of protein source you will feed your child. Make it a wise one.*
- *If you are a vegetarian, ensure that you are eating at least two different types of protein daily to ensure that all of the essential amino acids are absorbed.*
- *Be mindful of the amount of meat that your child is eating. It may be a great protein source, but it is also high in saturated fat and cholesterol.*
- *As the amino acids are important for aiding the neurotransmitters, ensure that your child is eating enough protein on a daily basis.*

VITAMINS & MINERALS

Vitamins

We have all heard the hype about vitamins, and how they are supposed to be good for our bodies. There are so many varieties of multi-vitamin supplements found in the supermarkets, drugstores and elsewhere that it can be very confusing as to which one to choose, if any.

When a child has a cold, the most common advice is "give them some vitamin C," but most parents don't know why. Many families mindlessly fall into the trap of giving their children a chewy multi-vitamin, which probably contains more sugar than vitamins.

To diffuse your confusion, I will explain what a vitamin is, and why it is important that we include all the main ones in the form of food in our family's diet every day. I will go into the different vitamins and the best sources, as well as what signs to look out for that indicate a possible deficiency.

A vitamin is an organic chemical compound that your body needs for normal functioning. Your body cannot produce vitamins so these need to come from your diet intake, however, we only need a small amount of each vitamin daily to keep us healthy.

There are 13 vitamins that are split into two categories:

- *Fat soluble*, which consists of vitamins A,D,E and K
- *Water soluble* vitamins B and C.

The *fat soluble vitamins* need fat in the body to help them be absorbed. If your child's diet is lacking in fat, then these fat soluble vitamins may not be absorbed properly, and potentially the body will show signs of deficiency. I am talking about the good fats here, and not the bad fats which is in most processed meals.

Once the vitamins are absorbed in the fat globules, they travel through the lymphatic system of the small intestines, and are then stored in the liver. The liver excretes these vitamins into the blood stream as, and when, needed.

With the *water soluble vitamins*, they dissolve in water; unlike the fat soluble vitamins, they are *not* stored in the body. Instead, they are absorbed from the food we eat, processed, and then discarded via urine, so we require a continuous daily supply in our diet.

Giving your children fruit or vegetables as a snack in-between meals will help maintain the right levels of the water soluble vitamins.

Let's discuss each vitamin to help you understand their importance, and which foods you should ensure that your child eats on a daily basis.

Vitamin A: This vitamin comes in two forms:

- an animal form called retinol which is found in meat, fish, eggs and milk
- the vegetarian form is a beta carotene which is found in orange foods such as carrots, sweet potatoes and peppers. The brighter the color, the more beta carotene it contains. The beta carotene version converts into vitamin A (in the liver) depending on how much you need.

Vitamin A is essential for all of the cells in the body, in particular the skin and membrane of the cell. It is known as an antioxidant, and supports the immune system.

You have to be careful not to intake too much vitamin A, as it is stored in the liver and can be toxic. This is very uncommon in food sources.

Poor night vision, frequent colds, infections and dry flaky skin have been linked to a deficiency in Vitamin A.[1]

B Vitamins: When we eat foods such as carbohydrates, the body needs B vitamins to help convert this food into the energy we need. As B vitamins are water soluble, we need them every day. Once they enter the body, they travel around doing its work, and then exits the body around 5 hours later.

There are several different B vitamins, and each has its own role in the body. B vitamins also play a big part in helping convert amino acids into the neurotransmitters in the brain.

- B1 (thiamine)—Thiamin helps to convert glucose into energy and has a role in nerve function. If your children are not getting enough thiamine in their diet, they may feel weak and tired.[2] Whole grains, liver, milk, eggs, legumes are all high in vitamin B1.
- B2 (riboflavin)—Riboflavin is involved in energy production, body growth and red blood cell production, and it helps vision and skin health. Deficiency can show up as lip sores, sore throat or even anemia.[3] Dairy, eggs, green leafy vegetables, legumes and nuts are high in B2.
- B3 (niacin)—Niacin is also involved in energy production and helps keep the skin, nervous system and digestive system healthy. Deficiency can show up as digestive issues, inflamed skin or skin rashes.[4] Dairy products, cereals, fish, legumes and nuts are high in B3.
- B5 (pantothenic acid)—Pantothenic acid is needed to produce red blood cells. Deficiency can show up as headaches and fatigue. Good sources of B5 are eggs, dairy, nuts and whole grains.
- B6 (pyridoxine)—Pyridoxine is needed to break down protein and carbohydrates. It helps the formation of red blood cells, certain brain chemicals, and it makes antibodies to fight off infections. Deficiency can show up as coordination problems.[5] Avocado, banana, nuts, meat and whole grains are high in B6.

- B7 (biotin)—Biotin is needed to break down protein and carbohydrates. It also helps the body make hormones. Good sources of B7 are eggs, dairy, lean meats, nuts and whole grains.
- B12 (Vitamin B12)—is needed for metabolism and for the body's growth and development. Deficiency shows as anemia, weakness and loss of balance.[6] B12 is naturally found in animal foods; it is also found in nutritional yeast.
- Folate—is needed to form red blood cells, which carry oxygen around the body. It is needed for synthesis of many of the neurotransmitters. Legumes and green leafy vegetables are high in folate.[7]

So, in general, B vitamins are found in whole foods like nuts, seeds, greens, fruit and whole grains. They are also found in eggs, fish, meat and dairy products. B vitamins are needed for energy, but they also power the brain. The first sign that you may be deficient in B vitamins is your lack of energy, lack of concentration, and low mood.

Ask yourself, what did you give your child for breakfast this morning? Is concentration an issue at school?

Vitamin C: This vitamin is needed to make energy and collagen, which makes your skin healthy and also keeps your arteries strong too. It is a great immune booster, and is known for its role in fighting colds and infections.

As we cannot produce vitamin C, and as it is a water soluble vitamin, it needs to be included in our daily diet intake. It is found in fruits and vegetables. Broccoli and strawberries are great sources and both have more vitamin C than oranges. Deficiency symptoms include frequent colds, infections, scurvy, bleeding gums and easy bruising.[8]

Vitamin D: Vitamin D is a fat soluble vitamin. It is produced in the skin in the presence of sunlight. If you have enough sun, then it converts the cholesterol in your body into vitamin D. Oily fish and eggs also provide vitamin D, but a little sunlight is the best source.[9]

If we look back in time, humans used to walk around with minimum clothing, and were outdoors for most of the day. As such, they were able to get the right amount of vitamin D. However, in the modern world today, most people do not spend enough time outside, and if we do, we are covered up, making it hard to absorb the required amount of sunlight.

If you are dark-skinned, it is even harder for you to ensure you get the right amounts of vitamin D as you have pigments that filter out the UV rays that trigger the production of vitamin D.

Vitamin D is the "sunshine vitamin," and on average we need around 15-30 minutes of exposure to the sun on a daily basis to help produce the right amount needed for our bodies.[10] Therefore, it is good for your children to take a stroll outside or sit outside in a park and eat lunch or a snack.

Vitamin D is needed to help the absorption of calcium, and therefore necessary for healthy bones and teeth. Recently, it was discovered that vitamin D is great at boosting the immune system.[11] It is also great for the health of your heart. *Get some Vitamin D and be happy!*

Vitamin E: Vitamin E is a fat soluble vitamin. It is an antioxidant, and it protects us from damage. Vitamin E is also needed for immune health and keeps our skin healthy too. Good sources of vitamin E are oily fish, nuts (especially walnuts), seeds and wheat germ. Easy bruising, slow wound healing, and dry skin are signs of vitamin E deficiency.[12]

Vitamin K: This is also a fat soluble vitamin. This forgotten vitamin is made by the bacteria in the gut. It is essential for the blood clotting, and is often given to newborn babies. Recent evidence has shown that vitamin K is important in a newborn's formation; having enough vitamin K will help fix minerals into the newborn making them stronger. Vitamin K is found in leafy green vegetables, and deficiency can lead to bruising, and even in rare cases hemorrhaging. As most of vitamin K is made in the gut, it is very important to have good gut flora.[13]

Minerals

The body requires many minerals. These essential minerals are divided up into two groups: macro minerals and trace minerals. Both groups of minerals are equally important, however, trace minerals are needed in smaller amounts.

Let's go into each one to help you understand their importance.

Calcium: Calcium is essential for healthy bones and teeth, as calcium is the main component of them. Most people think that giving their children dairy is the only option they have for calcium intake, however, there are some alternative options like almonds, pumpkin seeds and green vegetables. You need to bear in mind that vitamin D and magnesium rich foods are also important to help make the absorption process more efficient. Signs to look out for that may indicate calcium deficiency are muscle cramps, joint pain and tooth decay.[14-15]

Chromium: Chromium makes insulin which is the hormone that controls blood sugar. Chromium is found in whole foods, nuts, seeds, beans, fruits and vegetables. Refined foods such as white rice and white pasta have had most of the chromium wiped out.[16]

When your child eats a treat containing sugar, their blood sugar level goes up and insulin is released, this uses up chromium. If your child's diet is mainly made up of refined foods, then they are not getting enough chromium in the first place.

They may experience symptoms like irritability, mood swings, and without effective blood sugar control your child could have consistent sugar cravings.

Iron: In red blood cells, hemoglobin fixes iron with oxygen, and thereby helps transport the oxygen around the body. If we don't have enough iron in our bodies, then the oxygen will not be transported efficiently, and we will have a low hemoglobin count. This is known as anemia and shows up as a person looking pale, being tired and lethargic.[17] Iron is found in red meat, eggs, beans, lentils, nuts and seeds. Vitamin C helps with the absorption of iron. So, *if your child is having eggs for breakfast, then add some orange segments to help with the iron absorption.*

Magnesium: This mineral is commonly known as a muscle relaxant, and helps bone formation along with calcium and vitamin D. If children find it difficult relaxing, sleeping or staying asleep then they probably need more magnesium in their diet. Good sources of magnesium are green leafy vegetables, nuts and seeds, specifically pumpkin and sunflower seeds. We use magnesium as a helping hand when my children are constipated.

Selenium: Selenium is an antioxidant, and helps boost the immune system along with protecting us from free radicals and other nasties. A deficiency in selenium makes children prone to infections.[18] Selenium is found in seafood, seaweed, seeds, sesame seeds and brazil nuts.

Zinc: I love zinc! This is my go to mineral on the first signs of a cold. Zinc is necessary for immunity, growth and energy production.[19] Deficiency normally shows up as little white spots on finger nails. Foods that are high in zinc are nuts, seeds, beans, eggs, meat and fish.

Vitamin & Minerals questions & answers

As a vegetarian, are there certain vitamins and minerals I would get more easily from a meat diet, so I need to make a conscious effort to eat food that will contains these? For example, I understand that anemia is more common in vegetarians.

When you eat a varied diet, you should be absorbing all the necessary vitamins and minerals. With Vitamin B12, the majority is found in animal meat, however, spirulina and algae are both good vegetarian sources of vitamin B12. If you try adding spirulina to your children's smoothie, that will help with levels. Algae can be found in a health food shops.

If you can get all your vitamins from food, are supplements needed?

There is a time lag between the time the fruit and vegetables are picked, when they reach the shops, and then when you purchase them. Therefore, the nutrient levels may be lower than if we get them straight from the farm. Also, the soil may be missing the ideal levels of trace minerals. It can be hard to ensure that you are fully covered for the daily amounts of each vitamin and mineral needed. If you are eating a well-balanced diet, then I don't think you need a supplement, but if you are eating processed meals or take-outs several times a week, then I would give your child a supplement. Speaking to a local nutritionist will help you decide on the levels needed.

I believe most of the vitamins and minerals come from fruit and vegetables. I heard that, some fruit and vegetables still have residue pesticides left on them. Can you please explain further?

The environmental Working Group (EWG) have a list of all the fruit and vegetables that have pesticide residual. The top twelve, known as the 'dirty dozen' are: apples, strawberries, grapes, celery, peaches, spinach, sweet bell pepper, nectarine, cucumber, cherry tomatoes, snap peas, and potatoes. In my opinion I would try and buy organic versions of these dirty dozen. You can find more details on:

http://www.ewg.org/foodnews/list.php

Vitamins & Minerals Summary

As your body cannot produce vitamins and minerals, it is important that you eat a variety of healthy foods to ensure that you absorb all the necessary ones required for optimal health.

FATS

Like every other food component we have discussed, when we consider fats, we are overwhelmed with too many options. There are several different types of fats, and they can be categorized into three different types: the *good, the not so good, and the bad.* We need fats; remember, even the tin man benefitted from some good old fashioned oil. However, the combination and volume of the fats that we are consuming is an area of concern.

The *good fats* are the essential fats. The essential fatty acids (EFA's) linolenic (omega 3) and linoleic acid (omega 6) need to be incorporated into your child's diet as these essential fats are found in the membrane of every cell in your child's body, and the quality of these cells are dependent on the source of fats. The better the quality, the more efficiently they can work in getting rid of carbon dioxide, which in turn makes it easier for nutrients and oxygen to get into the cells.

Essential fatty acids are like super heroes, as they help strengthen and build your child's immune system, they help absorb and transport vitamins around the body, and the best part is that they help support and nourish the nervous system and your child's brain function.

Both Omega 6 and Omega 3 are needed for optimal cell health. Your body cannot create essential fatty acids, so it is very important to include them in your child's daily diet. We need to aim for a diet consisting of a ratio of 1:1 (ratio of omega 6 to omega 3), however, the common American diet has a ratio of around 15:1.[1] This higher intake of Omega 6 in the diet can cause excess inflammation in the body. Medical research suggests that this imbalance ratio could be the cause of many illnesses.[1]

The main sources of Omega 3 are cold water fish, walnuts and flaxseeds. Like the other food groups, the **quality** of the food will also play a part in the amount of good fats it contains and is absorbed. For example, if we take fish, there is a difference in the quality and nutritional value between a farm raised fish and a fish raised in the wild. So, we need to be mindful of the source of the fish, and this will help us determine its value on our child. With fish, we also need to be aware of contaminants such as mercury levels. Therefore, eating fish every day could potentially be toxic.

Omega 6 can be found in numerous foods such as nuts, seeds and their oils. Refined oils such as soy and canola are used in many processed foods and packaged foods. It is no wonder why the ratio of Omega 6 to Omega 3 is off balance. If the standard diet is full of fast food and packaged snacks, then it's very easy to overdo on Omega 6, which leads to inflammation.

If your child has dry skin, cracked lips, frequent colds and allergies, then it may be a good idea to increase the amount of essential fats in your child's diet. Try to incorporate more Omega 3 fats and be mindful of the amount of pro inflammatory Omega 6 that your child may be consuming.

Saturated fats fall in the *not so good* category. Saturated fats are needed in our diet, but there is a reason I have classed it in the not so good category. If excessive amounts are consumed daily, then this can have a negative effect on your children's health.

Saturated fats are not essential, which means the body can manufacture them, however, they help the fat soluble vitamins such as A, D, E and K to be absorbed in the body. They also provide building blocks for cell membranes.

Children need fat for energy and growth so it is important to include foods that have saturated fat in their diet. However, they do not need excessive amounts on a regular basis!

Saturated fats are more commonly found in animal sources such as meat, eggs and dairy products. They can also be found in coconut and palm oils.

A diet high in animal meat and dairy products will lead to a high level of saturated fats. This can become a problem if your child is eating meat daily. Eating excessive amounts of saturated fats in their diet can have negative effects on their health.[2]

Finally, trans fats and partially hydrogenated fats are the *bad ones*. When trans fats are manufactured, they go through a process where hydrogen is added to vegetable oil, which causes the oil to become solid at room temperature. This process messes with the fat molecules, and the body cannot recognize it as food. These unrecognizable fat molecules can be a significant cause of inflammation.

Trans fats increase your cholesterol, they can clog attires, and they are one of the components that is the leading cause to the obesity problem we are faced with today.[3] Again, relying on fast food and packaged foods is not helping your child!

The reason why manufacturers use partially hydrogenated oil is that it gives food a longer shelf life. Some restaurants use partially hydrogenated vegetable oil in their deep fryers as it can be used over and over again. So, when people say fat makes you fat, it is this "bad" fat that we need to be careful of.[4]

Stay away from margarine, commercial cooking sprays, and heavily processed vegetable oils such as corn and canola. Look at labels to see if it contains hydrogenated vegetable oil. Also, any food that has a long shelf life such as a muffin that expires in six months probably contains either hydrogenated vegetable oil or trans fats.

I know it can be very easy in our busy everyday lives to rely on fast foods and ready-to-eat packaged snacks, but these '*bad*' fats interfere with the brain's use of the '*good*' fats. The brain will not receive the right quantity of fats in order to function properly.

One thing to bear in mind is that, in the United States, any product that contains less than 0.5gms of trans fat in a serving can be labeled as zero trans fats. This hidden trans-fat can add up especially if you are eating several servings. For example, a packet of chips may say it 'contains five servings' but how many times have you seen your child eat more than one serving?[5]

Fat plays an important role in our overall health. We need it for our cell membranes, and we also need it to absorb the fat soluble vitamins. The appearance of your hair and skin, for example, can be improved by including the '*good*' fats in your diet. However, excessive amounts of fats such as Omega 6, saturated and trans fats can lead to inflammation in your child's body, which unfortunately is the starting point of many serious illnesses as they grow older.

It is important to include as much of the essential fats in your child's diet in the form of Omega 3 foods such as nuts, seeds, and oily fish. You need to keep saturated fats to a minimum such as eggs, meat and dairy and avoid trans fats including hydrogenated oils like processed foods, frozen meals and most packaged snacks.

When cooking, choose olive oil (use low heat), sesame, coconut oil and grape seed oil.

Fats questions & answers

Can I give my child fish oil?

Yes, you need to choose a high quality one, that has had the toxins filtered from it.

My family likes sausages, burgers, roasted chicken, which are all high in fat. Can you suggest any healthier alternatives?

There are many ranges and makes of sausages, burgers, and roasted chicken. If you are buying meat from an organic, antibiotic free, grass fed animal, then the quality and nutritional value will be higher than if you get a burger from a fast food place. Eating heavy meat every day is not good so I would limit it to every other day, and choose the high end meat when you can afford it. On the other days, try vegetarian meals or oily fish which is high in Omega 3.

What do you cook with?

We use olive oil and coconut oil. Coconut oil is high in saturated fats, which we need to absorb the fat soluble vitamins. As coconut oil is medium chained fats, it is easier to digest.

My child is overweight, shall I reduce her fat intake?

I would need to look at her full diet. There are other foods that make people fat, one being sugar. High fructose corn syrup (HFCS) is in many foods that children eat, and I believe this is the main contributing factor in weight gain. Please look at her sugar content first. If she is eating a lot of foods with HFCS, then please reduce these first. We need saturated fat to absorb the fat soluble vitamins, and we need the essential fats for brain, tissue and cell health.

If there has not be any improvement with her weight gain after you have cut out HFCS, then I would look at her fat intake.

Fats Summary

- *Your child needs saturated fats to help absorb the fat soluble vitamins. However, be mindful of the amount that is consumed, as too much saturated fats can lead to an increase in cholesterol levels.*
- *Essential Fatty Acid's are important for brain health. You should aim for a ratio of 1:1 of Omega 6: Omega 3.*
- *Avoid trans fats and hydrogenated oils, as these are damaging in that they can cause inflammation, and deplete the essential fatty acids in the brain.*

DRINKS

Water

Water is essential to your child's health. It makes up about 70% of their body and about 80% of their brain.[1-2] Water helps nutrients flow into the cells and wastes flow out of them. It stops the lymphatic system from getting sluggish, which is important as the lymphatic system is part of the immune system and helps fight infections. Water helps you digest food, and helps avoid constipation. It helps get rid of waste in the form of stools. Water helps the kidney function better, and gets rid of waste in the form of urine. So, *you can see how important water is.*

Your children will lose water through sweat, urine and perspiration. Therefore, it is very important that your child consumes enough water daily not only to help with the general functioning of the body, but also to help replenish what is lost.

Signs that your child is not getting enough water are dry lips and skin, eyes are sunken, and urine is dark. One way to help teach your child the importance of water is to get them to check the color of their urine. Explain to them that dark means they are not drinking enough water, and that pale yellow means they are drinking enough.

My kids have been doing this since they were potty trained. They used to tell me the color each time but thankfully they now only tell me when it's dark, which is very rare as my children drink water like a fish. Another way to get your children to drink more water is to have it available. You have heard of the saying "out of sight, out of mind." If it is the only option they have, then they are more likely to drink it. Children tend to imitate their parents doings, so if they see you drinking lots of water, they will too.

An added point about the quality of water; a glass of tap water may contain toxins in the form of heavy metals, pesticides and solvents.[3] Chlorine is added to help filter away some of these toxins, but chlorine had also been known to kill away the intestinal flora. This is not good for gut health. We will be discussing gut health later in the digestion chapter. Plastic bottled water is another option but they also can cause problems. Most plastic bottles are made of toxins including BPA which is a hormone disrupter. The safer options are glass bottles or a water filter. With a water filter, there are many types available from attaching it to the mains so all water is filtered, or by getting a stand-alone water filter which will filter the tap water and makes it safer to drink.

As water is as vitally important as nutrient dense food, it is essential that your kids are drinking enough safe, clean water daily to keep them healthy.

Sports Drinks

Parents often say to me, "The kids do so many activities and I need to give them something more than water". They further justify their reasoning for giving a sports drink by adding that their children do "intensive training."

Sports drinks, such as Gatorade replace the water and electrolytes that are lost during sweating. They contain carbohydrates, minerals, electrolytes and flavoring. So, on the surface, yes they do the job for replacing all that is lost in the "intensive training." However, these drinks contain large amounts of sugar (around 20g) and if drunk regularly could contribute to childhood illnesses such as obesity. In the sugar chapter, I have gone into depth on the effects that sugar has on our bodies and our health.

I looked into healthier options also. When my children have been doing general sports or are out in the sun too long, I give them a shot of coconut water. Fresh coconut water is one of the richest natural sources of electrolytes and can be used to prevent dehydration.[4] It is definitely a healthier option than Gatorade.

So, to conclude, I suggest if your child is doing less than 30 minutes of exercise/sports then water is enough to hydrate them. If they are exercising or doing sports for more than 60 minutes, then coconut water will help to hydrate them and replenish the electrolytes lost. However, if you feel that they are training harder and sweating more, then add a pinch of Himalayan salt to the glass of coconut water.

Fizzy carbonated drinks

I am shocked each time I see a child drinking soda. I have seen children as young as 3-years-old drinking from a bottle of some sort of fizzy drink. *I wonder if their parents know what is in these drinks*? The main ingredients are either sugar or high fructose corn syrup.

The body handles fructose differently. When fructose hits the body, it *doesn't* send a signal to the pancreas to release insulin. So, this fructose is not used as fuel but instead the fructose goes straight to the liver where it is known to potently stimulate lipogenesis (the production of fats).

When the fructose hits the liver, the liver is consumed with 100% of the burden to break down this fructose. The fructose is converted to fat, and it starts to build up on the liver and other tissues as body fat; typically the abdominal.[5-7] If your child continues to drink fizzy drinks, then slowly but surely, their liver will get fatty and they will become overweight.

With 1 in 4 children in America being overweight,[8] I wonder how many of them are drinking fizzy drinks on a regular basis.

Drinks questions & answers

My children don't like just drinking water, what can I do?

There are many options, but fruit-induced water has been popular amongst my little fussy clients. You take a jug of water and put in some fruit slices and let it sit overnight. You can choose strawberries, oranges, or even cucumber. It gives the water a subtle flavor and the children will love it.

I used to drink Coca-Cola when I was a child, and I am not overweight.

The problem is that the number of foods and drinks available in the supermarket has grown exponentially since you were a child. Also, prior to 1980, most foods and drinks had sugar, which was bad but not as detrimental to the body as high fructose corn syrup (HFCS). After the 1980's, most companies replaced sugar with HFCS as it was cheaper and sweeter. The effect of HFCS is that it goes straight to the liver and turns into fat. So, if your child is drinking several cans per week, this is going to lead to a weight problem.

What's your view on fruit juice?

When you drink the fruit juice, the sugar will cause your blood sugar to rise quickly. I don't recommend you giving your child fruit juices regularly. Eating fruit is different, as the fibre in the fruit helps slow down the release of sugar.

Drinks Summary

- *Water should be the first drink children are offered, as 70% of the body is made up of water.*
- *If your child is doing sports, be mindful of the sports drinks, as they are more than likely to contain sugar in one form or another.*
- *If you only have water in your home, then your children are less likely to ask for, or expect anything else.*

PART II
ESSENTIAL COMPONENTS OF A HEALTHY BODY

THE DIGESTIVE SYSTEM

Many adults I know complain about their digestive system, whether it's bloating, gas, or a full blown digestive disorder. Most of them are unaware how allergies, arthritis, autoimmune disease, rashes, acne, chronic fatigue, and even mood disorders can often be linked to problems with the gut. I asked them, "*If you could go back in time and change your diet to avoid this pain, would you*?" They all said yes.

So, why don't we do something today to ensure that our children's digestive system is not pushed to its limits, and they are given a chance to avoid some of the same issues that we adults face.

The digestive system runs from your mouth to your anus, and contains various parts in-between. It is a very complex internal system, and most of us do not give it much credit on how hard it needs to work.

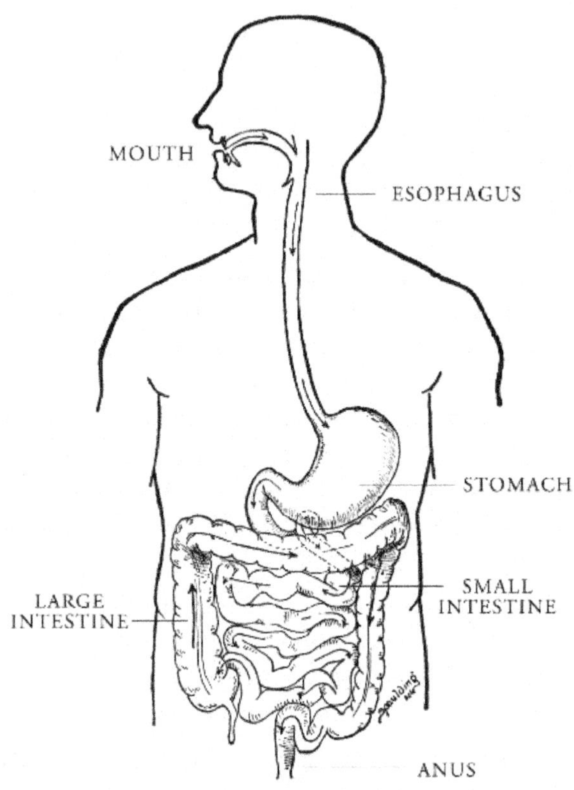

The digestive system helps us obtain nutrients from the food we eat and transfers it into our blood. It also helps us eliminate any waste and transports it out via poop!

Another big job that your digestive system has is that it contains a majority of your immune system. Around 70% of the immune system is found in the gut.[1]

This is a fascinating topic in itself, and we will go into this area in more detail later in the immune system chapter on how the immune system and gut are interrelated.

How does our food travel through the digestive system?

First, the food is broken down in the mouth by chewing. Saliva, which contain enzymes, helps the process and the food is broken down into small pieces.

The food molecules enter the stomach, and here the stomach acid and more enzymes further aide this breaking down process. This produces chyme.

The chyme makes its way to the intestines, where the enzymes from the gall bladder and pancreas further break it down to enable your body to extract the nutrients.

The good stuff (i.e. the nutrients) are transported to the blood stream, and the bad stuff (i.e. the poop) is transported out of the body.

How can you tell if your child's digestive system is working well?

Your child should be passing one to three well-formed stools per day.[2] These should look like a long sausage, and your child should not have to force out the motion. If the stools are small pellets or hard to pass, this could indicate your child is not eating enough fibre or drinking enough water. The poop should be mid brown, soft and easy to pass. Any pain or discomfort could be an indicator that your child's digestive system is not working as well as it should. Another indicator is the time your child spends passing the stool; if they are in the bathroom for a long time, I suggest you look into why. As the detective that I am, I can tell a lot when I go to people's houses and find a pile of magazines in the bathroom!

It all begins with chewing

So, we now know that good digestion has to start with chewing. How many children eat on-the-go and in-between activities? Or, they may gobble down breakfast in a hurry so they are not late for school. Do you think this food has been broken down into the right consistency for the stomach to do its job correctly? Or, do you think the child is swallowing bigger chunks of food?

Good chewing needs to be instilled in your child from day one. *Why do we give babies mush to eat*? It's the right consistency for them to start their digestion properly as they don't have teeth.

It is very hard for the child, especially when we as parents keep saying "hurry up." They need to be taught how to chew. We still have days when I have to remind my children to slow down. I know it can be time-consuming and sometimes very frustrating, but we owe it to our kids to start them off on the right foot.

A simple way to get saliva, stomach acid and enzymes ready and gearing to do its job is by getting the kids involved in laying the table. They will smell and see the food they breathe in, and become excited about the meal. This triggers the brain to release all the necessary "digestive busters" to help digest the food. Sitting down and eating a meal as a family is very powerful. Not only are you spending quality time together, but it also helps us slow down to fully engage and enjoy our meal slowly!

Food for Thought...If your child is eating a meal in-between activities and is rushed because you are running late, do you think they are chewing their food? Are they starting the digestion process off on a good foot?

Now, let's look at some typical foods your child might eat. I want you to think about your digestive system and the process of chewing. Would you think these foods are easy or hard to digest? Do you believe that your child is chewing these foods down to mush, or swallowing bigger parts?

- Cereal
- Porridge
- Toast
- Crackers or chips
- Fruit
- Veggie sticks
- Smoothies
- Yogurt
- Pizza
- Sandwiches
- Burgers
- Fish/ Chicken
- Steak
- Lentils/ Beans

The list can go on and on. I hope you now understand the importance of chewing, and how good digestion begins here. It is very easy to gulp down food, but by giving children time to eat, it can help them chew and set the right foundation for good digestion.

Stomach

The stomach is a hollow organ that holds food while it is being mixed with enzymes and stomach acid that continue the process of breaking down food into smaller components. If your child is not chewing their food properly, the stomach has to work harder to dissolve the food in the right consistency. Remember, the stomach does not have teeth to help breakdown the food quicker. When the contents of the stomach are sufficiently processed, they are released into the small intestine.

Small Intestine

The intestine, also known as the colon, is the longest part of the digestive system. If you stretch it completely out, it would cover the surface of a tennis court. The food enters the intestine from the stomach, where it is further broken down by enzymes from the pancreas and bile from the liver.

In the intestine, the food is fully digested, and nutrients are absorbed through villi (hundreds of small finger like folds). These villi are located in the intestinal wall, and are about one cell layer thick. Even though the villi are very small, they are responsible for producing digestive enzymes, absorbing nutrients, and blocking the absorption of harmful substances. So, it is very important to ensure that the villi does not get damaged.

The small intestine is made up of three parts: duodenum which is responsible for the continuous breaking down process, and the jejunum and ileum are responsible for absorption of nutrients into the blood stream. A lot of things go on in the intestine!

My beautiful son, who does not have a gall bladder, was in a lot of pain a few months after his liver transplant. Food would hit the intestine and there was no bile there to help further break it down. This causes a lot of tummy cramps. Other times, the bile would flow into the intestine and there was no food there, so he was in pain then too. By ensuring he was given easy to digest foods and eliminate foods that were causing problems, I was able to help regulate the bile so it flowed more efficiently. Thankfully, now, it all seems to be in sync with each other.

So, why are there so many digestive problems out there? One of the main starting points is that this villi becomes damaged. Some children may not be able to tolerate certain foods such as dairy, gluten or even carrots. The intolerance may not be life threatening but is enough to irritate the gut, and this will eventually damage the gut lining and the villi.[3] The gut will gradually lose its ability to distinguish between nutrients and harmful substances.

As the villi gets damaged, the barrier between the

inside and outside world becomes damaged as well. *A leaky gut* is the technical name for the damage. Your child could potentially become allergic to foods they may have previously been able to digest. The reason for this is that the villi has been damaged and the gut lining has become irritated, so some foods may just be harder to digest now.

To look at this in another way, if the gut lining is not optimal, your child could experience an *allergic reaction* to certain foods. This may show up as a rash or tummy ache. When the gut gets stronger, these allergic foods may actually become tolerable.

This was the case with my son. When he had strawberries for the first time, his arms became itchy. We stopped giving strawberries to him and reintroduced it every 6 months. This went on for 5 years. Now, he can eat strawberries happily with no allergic reaction. Unfortunately, my son had negative reactions to many foods including carrots, apples, and hummus. It was easy for us to spot these reactions as I followed a very specific weaning guide, and I was very mindful of each food we tried, and was on the lookout for any possible reactions.

Another indication of the gut lining being damaged is by looking at its link with the immune system. As most of the immune system lies in the gut, damage will affect the child's immunity. The immune system will think it is under attack from masses of invaders and it will become overactive, and consequently begin producing inflammation throughout your child's body. This could show up as a fever, cold, or flu-like symptoms.

I believe that your child's constant colds or the flu could potentially be initiated by the damaged lining in the gut? What could have damaged the gut lining? Antibiotics, foods that are causing irritation to the gut, and even a toxin such as sugar.

Large Intestine

That was deep, right! Okay, let's carry on with the digestive system. We will assume that there is no damage to the gut lining, and the small intestine does its job properly. Nutrients are absorbed and transported in the blood stream and the leftover-food residue liquid, bacteria and fibre passes through the small intestine into the large intestine.

The large intestine is small compared to the small intestine. It is about five feet long. Its job is to absorb the water and any further nutrients from the chyme and form the stool (poop). If the chyme passes through the large intestine too quickly, then the water is not absorbed and you end up with diarrhea. If the stool sits in the large intestine for too long, it becomes dry and hard to pass, which leads to constipation.

Anus

The final part of the digestive system is the anus. The stool travels from the large intestine through the rectum, and out of the anus.

That is the digestive system. It is very complex, and it is responsible for the majority of our well-being. A simple invader, whether it is a food you are allergic to, toxins, sugar or medication, can all impact the functioning of the gut lining and hence lead to complications. The Gut is where most of the immune system lies, so a damaged gut will affect your ability to fight infections. The gut also has a connection with the brain. We will discuss the gut-brain connection later in the brain chapter.

I am hoping that all of this information has not frightened you, but rather it has enlightened and made a positive impact on you. Being mindful of food reactions is very important for the health of the gut. I hope that you will be more mindful of what you feed your children, and learn to recognize these reaction signs, if any.

Gut Bacteria

Another major topic to discus in this chapter is all about gut bacteria. This seems to be the new buzz word, and the general public is becoming aware of the importance that gut bacteria plays in their health. They are trying hard to add the good bacteria into their daily diet in the form of probiotics; many people choose probiotic yogurts in the market. Through clever marketing, these yogurts are popular but they have limited probiotics, and instead most often these yogurts contain a high percentage of sugar which defeats the purpose as the bad bacteria (which is also present in the gut) feed off this sugar.

What is Bacteria?

Within our digestive system, there are over 100 trillion microbiota (bacteria) cells.[4] Gut flora is a general name for the microbiota (bacteria), and a good balance of gut flora is essential for healthy digestion. Billions of bacteria reside in the mouth, however, the stomach has a far lesser amount because of the high acid content that prohibits their growth. The small intestine has many billions of bacteria, but the majority of the gut flora inhabit the large intestine i.e, the colon.

We all have a combination of good and bad bacteria in our gut. The *good* bacteria offers us protective and nutritive properties, whereas the *bad* bacteria can cause acute or chronic illness. We need to ensure that we have an abundance of the good bacteria, and a limited amount of the bad bacteria.

History of Bacteria

Where do we get the bacteria from? Unfortunately, it all starts with our mom. When our mother has an abundance of good bacteria in her gut, this travels into other parts of the body including the vagina. When a baby is born and travels through the birth canal, the baby swallows bacteria, which becomes their gut flora.[5-6] The baby is further exposed to bacteria in breast milk, when sucking nipples, fingers and toes. With every breath and touch, bacteria enters the baby's body. Within a few days, the digestive system is occupied by billions of microbes.

If the baby is unable to properly colonize friendly flora, they become colicky, irritable and may have gas pains and nappy rash.[7-9] Babies who don't develop the right balance of beneficial bacteria are more susceptible to allergies, asthma and eczema.

If you had a caesarian, and/or bottle fed your child, then they may not have been given the best opportunity to gather the right bacteria. I would supplement them with a baby friendly probiotic with the bifidobacteria infantis strain. Your local health care shop will be able to assist in this. Good quality probiotics will be found in the refrigerated section.

The colonization structure we set up in infancy continue to be present throughout our entire lives. Therefore, it is important to give our newborns the best opportunities to maximize their gut flora from an infant age.

Why is gut flora important?

The gut flora helps the body digest certain foods that the stomach and intestine were unable to break down and digest. It helps the production of vitamin K and B vitamins.[10] Vitamin K is needed for proper blood clotting, and B vitamins power the brain. So, if the gut flora is not optimal, then your child may bruise easily or they may show signs of brain fog, irritability or even lack of concentration. Gut flora produces disease-fighting antibodies, which help boost the immune system.[11] Thus, it is very important that we have optimal good bacteria in our gut.

How do the good guys get taken over by the bad ones?

There are both good and bad bacteria in the gut. Some things will enhance the good, and others will feed the bad.

Antibiotics will wipe out the good guys.[12] I know many parents who opt to give their children one antibiotic after another to help with an ear infection or fever. The sad thing is that the good bacteria is wiped out in the process, and it will take around two to four weeks to repopulate. During this time, there is a window of opportunity for pathogens to establish new territories in the gut. *Once in, it is hard to drive them out!* It is very common for children to be on several courses of antibiotics during their childhood, and this will damage the gut flora, and in the process the immune system will be compromised.

Can you see the pattern? If your child does need antibiotics, I would recommend introducing a good probiotic after the course is finished. This will help repopulate the good bacteria quicker, and hopefully before the pathogens take homage. (You will need to get this probiotic from a health food store as the majority of the commercial ones do not have the right strength and are high in sugar).

Sugar is another problem. The bad bacteria love sugar, and it feeds off it, and consequently grows in volume and again damages the gut flora. A bad diet full of sugary foods is also a contributing factor on depleting the good bacteria.

This problem can get out of hand. If the bad guys take over, or if they move into other areas of the gut, for example the small intestine, then the bad bacteria will start fermenting the food you digest, which will cause bloating, a feeling of fullness, and an over-production of gas. This is called small bowel bacterial overgrowth(SBO).

The only way to treat this is by using a non-absorbed antibiotic, which will reduce the bloating and overall symptoms associated with SBO. A high strength probiotic is usually prescribed and, in my opinion, we need to look at the reason why the bacteria went out of control in the first place and treat this. It could have been food allergies, over-consumption of processed foods, sugar, lack of digestive enzymes, parasites living in the gut, nutrient deficiency such as zinc or magnesium, or there could be heavy metal toxicity (does your child have a lot of fillings?). It is, therefore, important to personalize the treatment. We need to look carefully at the underlying causes and treat them.

An example to explain the importance of good gut flora...A life of a three-year-old.

The day begins with a sugar rich cereal, and for lunch mom makes some pasta with sauce. Snack is usually something from a packet; these simple carbohydrates become the norm for this busy mom. At preschool, there is a lot of tummy bugs and colds and the chances that your child picks up a bug is very high. This three-year-old ends up with a fever and a chesty cough. Mom takes the child to the doctor and a course of antibiotics is started. These antibiotics are taken for about 7 days, and during this time most, if not all, the friendly bacteria has been destroyed. This little child goes back to preschool with depleted good bacteria, and is back to eating her sugary cereals and packaged snacks. The bad bacteria (which does not get destroyed after the course of antibiotics and is nourished by a bad diet) is having a party and growing in numbers. As I mentioned before how the bad bacteria can cause acute or chronic illness. The story continues....

Leaky Gut

Leaky gut is a condition that occurs due to the development of gaps between the cells that make up the lining of your intestinal wall. All the above situations may, over time, end up causing these gaps. If your child continues to eat food that may be causing damage, then this can eventually break away the gut flora and then it may work its way through the gut lining and hence cause these gaps.

These tiny gaps allow substances such as undigested food and bacteria that should be kept within the digestive tract, to escape into the blood stream. Once the gut lining is broken, there will be a flow of toxic substances "leaking out" into the blood stream. This may cause an increase in inflammation. All this is largely influenced by the foods you choose to feed your children.

Signs of leaky gut

- diarrhea, constipation, gas or bloating
- Nutritional deficiencies
- Poor immune system; constant colds or coughs
- Find it hard to concentrate
- Overly tired
- Skin rashes; such as eczema
- Sugar cravings

How can we nourish…enhance the good bacteria to prevent leaky gut?

- Firstly, I would remove anything that is causing an issue in the gut. Look at your child's diet and see how much sugar, processed foods, hard to digest foods and such that they are eating. All these will impact the digestive system and affect the gut flora, so removing them will help heal the gut.
- I would look out for any reactions such as rashes, tummy pains, ear and nose mucus. I would try and figure out which foods are causing the reaction and also take these out of the diet. This will give the gut time to heal, as overloading it with reactive foods (allergy foods) will cause irritation in the gut and inflammation.
- Once you have identified the potential cause, you then need to increase the intake of good bacteria. You could start with natural yogurt. Unlike the probiotics, they will not stay in the gut, so it's important to continue eating it daily.

  Foods that are high in polyphenols are also recommended in healing the gut. They increase the number of beneficial bacteria, such as lactobacilli and bifidus. They also reduce disease-causing bacteria. Examples of foods that are rich in polyphenols are broccoli, celery, onions, almonds, cashew nuts, apples, blackberries, blueberries, and you could add basil, cinnamon and chives as seasoning. We have recently introduced fermented vegetables daily. They have increased probiotic content, they aide in digestion, and provide health-building enzymes. I personally noticed a difference in the way I felt within a few days. My daughter finds the taste a bit odd, but she must have found it helped as she openly accepts it now.

How to make fermented vegetables:

2 quart-sized mason jars

Fabric and an elastic band

Large mixing bowl

1 medium head of green cabbage or red cabbage

1 ½ tablespoons sea salt

- Clean and rinse everything thoroughly.
- Keep two large whole cabbage leaves aside for later. Cut out the core of the cabbage and slice the remaining cabbage thinly.
- Combine the cabbage and salt in the mixing bowl and start to massage the cabbage with your hands. As the cabbage begins to wilt, it should begin to release juices.
- Pack into the jars as tightly as possible and press down your whole cabbage leaves on top to hold it in and make a plug. There should be enough liquid so the cabbage is submerged. If it is not, mix 1 tsp salt with 2 tbsp water and add to the jar and then press down firmly. Cover with the fabric and elastic band.
- Place in the pantry and allow to ferment for 5-10 days. It should bubble and you will need to toss the cabbage daily. Taste it and sometimes it will be ready after 5 days, other times it may take 10 days. Once the fermenting process has been done, move it to the fridge to continue to ferment. You will be able to enjoy the veggies after a couple of days.

Finally, you could also include a good probiotic supplement. There are many on the market so ensure they are of high quality that include billions of lactobacilli and bifidus and it is age appropriate. These are usually refrigerated and found in the health food store.

- I would also consume high quality fish oil to further aide gut inflation. It has a cooling effect on the body.
- If the gut has gone through a lot of damage, I would add in glutamine and zinc to help repair the lining in your gut so it can resume its normal function. (Your local nutritionist or health food shop can help you with this).

Digestive System question & answers

My children always eat in a rush. What can I do to help them slow down?

We play a game "who can chew the food the longest?" I start counting and the child who is left chewing wins.

I had a caesarian and bottle fed my child. I am worried that their gut has not got the optimal level of good bacteria. What can I do?

First, please don't worry. I would introduce a probiotic daily and this will help populate the good bacteria. Your local health food shop will be able to advise you on the right one for your child, depending on their age. I would also introduce half a teaspoon of fermented vegetables twice a week. This will help strengthen the gut lining and also help populate the good bacteria. With children, in most cases, it does not take much time to resolve an issue, so I am confident that you will see a difference.

My child does not go to the bathroom every day. I am worried he is constipated.

First, I would ensure that he is drinking enough water and eating enough vegetables as this will help move things along. Without knowing his daily diet, I cannot comment on what he eats, but a diet full of processed meals and fast take-out foods will clog any one up. Highlight foods that may be causing problems with his digestion and try to omit these to see if that makes a difference. I am confident that changing elements of his diet and adding in vegetables and water, will help.

Digestive System Summary

The digestive system is very complex, and even if one part is less than optimal, this can cause a lot of health problems. I would advise you to re-read the chapter a couple of times to fully digest and understand the make-up of the digestive system, including what will strengthen it, or potentially weaken it.

BRAIN POWER

How to keep your child's brain healthy

For our children's optimal brain power, we need to ensure the following:

Their blood sugar is balanced. As we discussed in the carbohydrates section, balancing blood sugar is very important for our overall health. The brain is fuelled by the glucose that is converted from the carbohydrates that we eat. The right type of carbohydrates i.e., complex carbohydrates and the timing of how often you are consuming carbohydrates is very important. Your child should be eating three main meals with about two snacks in-between. This is why it is so important that your child starts the day with a healthy breakfast and that snacks are not full of sugar, as it will play havoc with their blood sugar.

A diet high in simple carbohydrates will cause the blood sugar to rise, and this can potentially cause hyperactivity (effect brain sensitivity). This sudden rush of sugar to the brain will soon be followed by a sudden crash from the sugar intake. If your child eats small amounts of complex carbohydrates often, then it will help keep the child's energy and concentration levels balanced. Adding protein will also help slow down the release of the glucose.

To *help you understand this further, remember the day when you were busy rushing out the door in the morning, and you did not have time to eat breakfast. Around 9:00am, you needed a boost so you reached out for caffeine and sugar. You missed lunch as you were busy working, and again reached for something quick and sugary. The kids arrive home from school and you are so hungry and your brain is foggy. Your tolerance level has dropped. Who gets the brunt of your mood? Your child! So, even for us parents, it is so important to start the day off with a healthy breakfast, and ensure that you are eating snacks to keep your blood sugar stable.*

1. Ensure that your children are eating enough foods that provide them with the right vitamins and minerals. As you read in the vitamins and minerals section, you can see that there are many vitamins and minerals needed for cognitive health. Ensure that your child has *at least* five portions of fruit and vegetables daily. In the diary section for younger children, I have set up a rainbow that will encourage children to eat a rainbow a day. This simple exercise has been very popular with my clients in that children have been asking to try different colored fruits and vegetables.

2. Avoiding anti nutrient foods will help give your child's brain some rest. Foods high in refined sugars, high fructose corn syrup, additives and damaged fats all have a negative impact on the brain. In some cases, they can damage the neurotransmitters and cause cellular damage to the brain.[1] As mentioned in the sugar section, too much sugar can deplete the dopamine receptors in the brain, and this can have a knock on effect with your child's mood. I go into more detail below on how nutrients affect the neurotransmitters.[2]
3. In the gut section, I explained how a damaged gut can have an impact on the absorption of nutrients. This lack of absorption can also impact your brain. There is a gut-brain relationship which I will go into, where you will be able to understand how important it is to be mindful of foods that your child may be allergic or intolerant to. These foods not only damage the gut, but through the gut-brain connection they also start to damage the brain.
4. Finally, to keep the brain healthy, you need to ensure it is fed the right fats. 60% of the brain is made up of fat, so you can see how important it is for the brain to consume the right fats.[3] As you read in the fats section, there are many types of fats and some are damaging. Unfortunately, most take-out meals people eat are made from these unhealthy fats. Some of the packaged snacks have the damaging oils too. It is therefore important to get the right fats into your child's diet intake. Eating foods

high in essentials fatty acids, mainly Omega 3 such as nuts, seeds, omega rich eggs and oily fish will help boost your child's intake of "good" fats.[3]

Neurotransmitters

We touched on this a little in the protein section on how neurotransmitters are made from amino acids. These amino acids are metabolized from the protein that we eat. The amino acids are not only needed for tissues, fiber, skin and hair, but they are also needed to make neurotransmitters. It's not as simple as upping your protein because turning amino acids into a neurotransmitter needs the right minerals, vitamins and oxygen. The main neurotransmitters that are likely to affect your child are serotonin, dopamine, adrenalin and GABA. Let's delve into each one.

Serotonin: Serotonin keeps us happy and improves our mood by banishing the blues. The amino acid tryptophan is needed to synthesis into serotonin. Tryptophan is found in many foods including cottage cheese, tofu, bananas, tuna, hazelnuts, chocolates, avocado and broccoli. Low serotonin levels cause problems with sleeping, make us sad, and in extreme cases cause aggressive behavior. Adequate levels of vitamin B1, B3, B6 and folic acid are needed to ensure that tryptophan is converted to serotonin.[4]

Dopamine: Dopamine is needed for healthy assertiveness and motivation. As we discussed earlier, sugar stimulates the dopamine receptors, and a diet full of sugar will start to destroy the receptors. The amino acid phenylalanine is needed to make the dopamine, and it requires a lot of fruits and vegetables to help with the production. Eggs, dairy, meat, legumes and nuts are high in phenylalanine. Tyrosine amino acid can also be used to manufacture dopamine. Tyrosine rich foods consist of almonds, avocados, pumpkin seeds, bananas and dairy.[5] There have been a few studies stating that children with ADHD have low levels of dopamine.[6-7]

Noradrenalin: This neurotransmitter is needed for motivation, alertness and concentration. Noradrenalin is needed to form new memories, and to shift them to long-term storage. Like dopamine, this neurotransmitter is formed through phenylalanine and tyrosine.

GABA: Gamma-Aminobutyric acid (GABA) helps the central nervous system function. The amino acids that synthesizes to GABA are taurine and glutamine. If the brain is lacking in GABA, then it will show up as a child who is irritable and hyper. GABA calms down the overexcited nervous system. Foods that can add to the production of GABA include lentils, bananas, whole wheat, eggs, broccoli and almonds.

As you can see now, several different types of foods are needed to help produce the neurotransmitters. The impact of having low levels of these neurotransmitters shows up negatively in children. Mainly, it shows up as a child being hyperactive, restless and with low concentration. Most of the amino acids need the right vitamins, minerals and oxygen to aide the production. If your child is eating a varied whole food diet, then they should be okay in achieving optimal protein, vitamin and mineral levels. However, as we have seen too many times, the average on-the-go American child has limited nutritious meals, and therefore certain elements like the neurotransmitters will be effected.

We are all aware of the neurons in the brain, however, we have millions of neurons in the gut lining as well. The enteric nervous system uses many of the same neurotransmitters as the central nervous system. For example, if we take serotonin, there is greater concentration of serotonin neurons in the gut than in the brain.[8]

Gut-Brain Connection

In the early embryo stage, the gut and brain came from the same tissue. During the fetal development, the tissue splits onto two parts; one becomes the central nervous system (cns), and the other becomes the enteric nervous system (ens), sometimes called the second brain. The cns is composed of the brain and spinal cord, and the ens is the intrinsic nervous system of the gastrointestinal system. These two connect via a nerve from the brain stem into the abdomen. This is the starting point of the gut-brain connection.

Have you noticed that when you are angry and stressed you may have stomach pain, or when you are nervous or excited you have butterflies in your stomach? If we are calm, the brain sends signals to release digestive enzymes which are needed to help digest your meal. The stomach will not show signs of irritation. On the flip side, if your gut is not in optimal condition, then whatever you eat, due to the damage, it will make you sad and anxious. We discussed many reasons in the gut chapter on how the gut may potentially get damaged.

Now, if you consider your child, have there been times when they were sick with a tummy bug and felt very sad? Are there days when your child is angry and they eat their food quickly, and then complain of a tummy ache? Another common problem is with little babies, have you wondered why that poor baby is crying all night? Maybe it's because their tummy is upset and they are sad, and the only way they can express it is through crying. Adding to this problem is that when they are upset and crying, the brain is not calm and the message to signal to the digestive system to release the digestive enzymes to help digest the food is altered. This can be a vicious cycle which many parents go through. A baby cannot distinguish the difference between the pain of hunger and the pain of a tummy ache. The mother keeps feeding the baby and soon after the baby poops and stops feeding, however, this constant feeding is the most likely reason for the tummy pains in the first place.

I believe that it is very important to ensure gut health is optimal and this will help with the brain too.

Concentration and Memory

As you can see, the health of the brain is very much dependent on what we eat. Not only will nourishing foods give us the boost of amino acids, vitamins and minerals that are needed, it will also help heal the gut. A diet lacking in nutrients leads to a foggy brain, and problems with concentration and memory.

Stabilizing the blood sugar by concentrating on complex carbohydrates and good protein along with loads of fruit and vegetables will help improve concentration and memory. The brain is getting constant fuel to help it function properly. There are certain foods that will enhance memory and concentration.

As we mentioned above, essential fatty acid (EFA's) is much needed as 60% of the brain is fat. Including oily fish, nuts and seeds will make a difference to your child's concentration and memory levels. Eggs are powerful too as they contain nutrients such as phosphatidyl choline and phosphatidyl serine which stimulate the brain chemical acetylcholine. Acetylcholine is involved in improving memory. GABA helps calm down an overexcited nervous system. Therefore, including the GABA foods will help with concentration.

If a child is eating a high sugar cereal for breakfast, sugary snack, processed lunch, another sugary snack after school and fast food take-out for dinner, you can see that this will not be optimal for all the cells, nerves, and chemicals in the brain.

Mood and Behavior

Children, like adults, have bad days and they can get angry and sad; unfortunately, they may not express their feelings in an optimal way. It could be as simple as hunger which is causing the change in behavior (blood sugar problems) or it could be that they lack key nutrients.

A few years ago, we saw a child in the clinic who was very sad with life. The mother had tried everything, but it was not making any difference. After some testing, the results showed that she was lacking key "brain" nutrients such as zinc and magnesium. As the case was severe, supplements were advised and the girl was much better after a few weeks. This is a severe case but I wanted you to see how getting the right nutrients can make such a difference in the way you feel.

The main nutrients linked to mood and behavior are vitamins B3, B6, B12, C, zinc, magnesium and essential fats.[9] You can see in the vitamin and minerals section which foods are high in these nutrients. Ensuring that the child has a good supply of these during the day will be one positive step towards helping your child improve their mood, behavior, and overall health.

Serotonin is the happy neurotransmitter and therefore following the advice from above will also help shift your child's mood.

The amino acid tryptophan is needed to synthesis into serotonin. Tryptophan is found in many foods including cottage cheese, tofu, bananas, tuna, hazelnuts, chocolates, avocado and broccoli.

It can be very unnerving to watch a child go through various emotions and behaviors, and feeling lost in what you can do to make a change. My daughter is 'spirited', she has a heart of gold, if she is behaving inappropriately at times, I take a step back to observe what is going on. Has she been eating her meals? Is something upsetting her? Has she been to the bathroom? Has she had a good night's sleep. Most times, it has been something that is easily fixable.

My daughter has spent her whole life watching her brother go in and out of the hospital. She never knew how to express her concerns, and she would usually try and act 'naughty' to get the attention that she felt was missing. As a mother, I can see the reason behind her behavior, but others may not see it. Through the help of great teachers along the way, we have been able to give her what she needs, and that is positive reinforcement. My daughter has shown a lot of improvement.

I will never forget the day when she shouted at the doctors for hurting her brother (they were trying to take blood). She went up to her brother and held him, and kept rubbing his forehead while holding one hand. So, to me, this is so much more important. Teaching children about compassion is often lacking, as many adults themselves are busy in their lives that they may not see that someone is in need. To me personally, I am grateful that my daughter has this skill because it is a powerful trait to have. With her 'spirited' personality, I believe she will do great things in her life.

So, to conclude in this section, many problems may be fixed by improving the child's diet, but when it comes to mood, behavior and emotions, I would look at what is going on with your child. Just by stepping back, taking a breath, and carefully observing your children can help you figure out if it's simple or if there is a hidden underlying problem.

Brain Power questions & answers

My child is always tired in the afternoon. What can I do to boost him up?

Most children have lunch, and then could go a few hours before their next meal. This could impact your child's blood sugar level and when it is low, people experience tiredness, irritability or even anger. I would try and ensure you have a healthy complex carbohydrate/protein snack ready for your child after school, and on the weekends ensure that they are eating every 2-3 hours to help stabilize blood sugar throughout the day.

My child finds it hard to sleep.

There could be a number of reasons why your child cannot sleep. He could be overstimulated from television, games, or sugar. he could be over-tired and then finds it hard to switch off, or he may need some help. Magnesium is great for 'calming' down the body. Taking a bath with Epsom salt will allow magnesium to enter the body through the skin. I would then add lavender to the feet and massage their body to release any tension. This should help calm him down and help with sleep.

IMMUNE SYSTEM

The immune system has probably the largest impact on a human's health. The cells of the immune system guard every component of the body, and they help defend us from invaders and cellular damage. As the cells of the immune system are in the blood stream and in our lymph nodes (which are located all over the body), they have the ability to quickly reach an invader as and when necessary. The defending cells will bind to the target, and wait for other cells to come along and remove it.

The immune system relies on the fact that the body has strong barriers in place between the inside and outside world. The most common barrier is the skin, however, most people are unaware that the intestinal tract acts like a barrier too.[1]

Let's look at an example with the skin. If your child has a cut on their finger, the immune system is triggered, as the cut is breaking the barrier between the inside and outside of the body. The finger becomes red and inflamed, this is the immune cells getting to work. They go to the site to attack and destroy the invaders, and then clean up the mess. This is when inflammation can be positive, however, it's a different story when something manages to get through the gut barrier.

70% of the immune system cells are found in the intestinal tract.[2] Your intestinal tract comes into contact with the largest amount and number of different molecules and organisms in the form of food. The gut has to figure out which molecules are bad for your child (the invaders), and it also needs to be able to absorb the nutrients from the good molecules in order to survive. In an ideal world, your child's intestinal tract will be optimal and be able to absorb the beneficial nutrients, and be able to excrete the not-so healthy organisms and molecules out of the body.[3]

However, as I explained in the digestion chapter, there are many ways the gut lining can get damaged, and in some cases it causes a leaky gut. If your child has a leaky gut, not only do the toxins enter their blood stream but the body will also find it hard to absorb vitamins, minerals and other nutrients from the food that your child eats.[4]

These toxins that enter the blood stream via the leaky gut signal the immune system to wake up and get to work. The immune system responds with inflammation. The immune system will become confused with what is invaders and what is not. If the leaky gut is not healed then, over time, the immune system can become overburdened and these inflammatory triggers travel through your blood and can start affecting nerves, organs, tissues and muscles.[5]

So, how does this affect your child?

If your child is eating a lot of foods that irritate their gut, then slowly the gut lining will become damaged. This leads to inflammation and the immune system will be overworked, and it will not know which way to go.

It's like a family with five children. The children are throwing toys all around the room. The parents can get to one child at a time, and that leaves three still busy destroying the house. Then, the parents go get another child and while they do that, the other two are released. This goes on and on. What happens next? The parents get tired and the house is a big mess. This is similar to what happens inside the body with the immune system. The immune system is busy trying to fight all the foreign particles and slowly and if a change is not made, then the inflammation keeps getting fueled and the immune system gets weaker.

How can you tell if your child has a not so optimal immune system?

Your child may take days to recover from a cold, they may be off sick with one bug after another. Or, they may be overly tired. I see this all the time at school, and some of these poor kids are then given antibiotics to help them with the illness BUT we know what antibiotics do, they destroy the gut flora. What happens when we have low gut flora? The bad guys take over. Then the bad guys start invading areas they shouldn't, and the cycle goes on and on.

This is a big thing in our home. Since my children

were babies, we have been giving them healthy probiotics and working on keeping their gut strong. As 70% of the immune system is in the gut, I believe this explains why they hardly get sick.

The Problem with Antibiotics

Many parents I know have opted for antibiotics to help fight one illness after another. From ear infections, to strep and even in some cases for the cold. It is very hard watching your child suffer, and be in pain, especially when they have a fever. Antibiotics can induce long-term damage to the gut flora.[6] When the good gut flora is wiped out, this gives the bad guys a chance to take over the territory. We learned in the digestion chapter how low good bacteria can have an effect on gut health. When the bad guys take over, it's very hard for the child's good flora to be optimal again without the help of a good probiotic.

When I see clients, I will look for what is causing the ear infection, strep, etc. Is it something they are eating that is causing a reaction, is it that they are not having enough high quality nutritional meals, the list goes on. The problem with most doctors is that they treat the symptom and not the cause. So, with the ear infection that has been treated with an antibiotic, the parent will go back to feeding the child the same way. I have seen this too many times when the poor child has reoccurring ear infections.

If the child was reacting to dairy and this was something the child had on a daily basis, then not only will the dairy keep causing ear infections, but the allergic reaction will keep irritating the gut. If the good flora is not there to help ease the allergic reaction, the effect of eating dairy will start causing the gut to leak.

I have seen this pattern happen far too many times, and the poor child ends up being sick more often than they should do.

In my opinion, if you give your child antibiotics, give them a good probiotic after the course has finished. This will help repopulate the good flora. If your child has regular illnesses, then I would look at their daily diet intake to see if there is something that may be causing a problem internally.

We need to break the cycle. How?

1. First, I would remove anything that is causing an issue in the gut. Look at your child's diet and see how much sugar, processed foods, hard to digest foods etc. they are eating. All of these will cause inflammation in the gut and put pressure on the immune system. The main culprits are gluten, dairy, and sugar.

2. Nutrients that have been demonstrated to be required for the immune system to function efficiently include essential amino acids, the essential fatty acids, vitamin A, folic acid, vitamin B6, vitamin B12, vitamin C, vitamin

D, vitamin E, Zinc.[7] Look over the vitamins chapter to get an idea of which foods are high in these nutrients and add them in to your child's diet.

3. I would add more anti-inflammatory foods to your children's diet.

   a. Increase their vegetable intake. Start with the ones they already eat and with each new one introduced, space it out to watch for any possible reactions. As mentioned in the gut chapter, my son reacted to certain foods over many years. Even now, whenever he eats a new food, I watch out for reactions, if there is one and I keep offering this vegetable to him, it will cause more damage than good.

   b. Fruits are also anti-inflammatory. The berries, apples, and grapes are good choices.

   c. Essential fatty acids are very calming to an inflamed body. We discussed these fats in the fats chapter, including oily fish, nuts, seeds can all help.

   d. Using turmeric, garlic, onions and ginger to cook with are super anti-inflammatory and flavorsome.

4. Increase the intake of good bacteria. You could start with natural yogurt. Unlike the probiotics, they will not stay in the gut so it's important to continue eating it daily.

5. Add in fermented vegetables. We have been adding these for a few months and I would recommend it for the entire family.

Immune System questions & answers

Come November each year, my child always gets one illness after the other, what shall I do?

I'd look at their diet and limit sugar, processed food and foods that might be causing a problem like gluten or dairy. Then, starting September, I would increase antioxidants foods such as vegetables, berries, fish, nuts, seeds, and cook with garlic and onions. These foods will boost the immune system as they heal the gut. This will give your child a "*protective*" layer so if someone is sick at school, they're less likely to catch it.

What is your opinion on antibiotics?

I personally do not agree with giving antibiotics for viral infections, however, for bacterial infections, I would. I recommend that you start with a good probiotic after the course has finished to help repopulate the good bacteria. If your child has several courses of antibiotics per year, then I would look at what is causing the problems. I treat the cause, and not the symptom.

What is your opinion on supplements?

I give my children supplements twice a week between September and February each year. Mainly zinc, vitamin C and vitamin D. This just gives them extra protection during the winter months. As for your child, you will need to see your local nutritionist so they can advise you on the proper dosages.

Immune System Summary

As 70% of the immune system resides in the gut, optimal gut health is very important to help improve immunity.

Nutrients such as vitamins and essential fatty acids are needed to ensure that the immune system functions efficiently.

Choosing an anti-inflammatory diet is highly encouraged.

PART III
ESSENTIAL COMPONENTS OF A HEALTHY SOUL

SOULFUL DIARY

I have kept a diary for most of my adult life. About 10 years ago, I added gratitude and desired feelings on how I wanted my day to go. This simple exercise has been powerful, and I have managed to achieve most of my dreams. By being grateful for what I have and by having a strong vision of my future has given me what I want.

My children have been keeping a diary for about a year, and it has been a positive addition to their day. It took a few weeks to implement the diary writing into their routine but both children have experienced a positive outcome. We have even began to notice a difference between the days they fill out the diary compared to the days they missed out on it.

Your child may find it difficult expressing themselves, or they may be happy to share everything going on in their life; either way I believe starting a practice of keeping a soulful diary will empower them in so many ways.

Some children find it difficult to express their feelings. If you watch a small child they often get frustrated as they struggle to find the right words needed to communicate how they feel. This frustration can result in tears, stomping their feet, or even acting out in rebellious ways.

As children get older and as they learn new words, they want to talk more and more about every little thing that comes to mind, or whatever goes on in their little lives. Sometimes, their little chats may not be at the most convenient time for their parents. The child may feel ignored and subsequently if this continues over and over again, the child may begin to suppress their feelings and stop sharing their feelings altogether.

I know a few adults that have experienced the feeling of being ignored when they were a child, and they also felt they were not given the space to express themselves freely. This may be the reason why they find it difficult communicating to friends and family members even now as an adult.

On the other hand, some children are eager to share everything and will not stop until someone has listened to what they have to say. They are enthusiastically excited, and at times, however, it may be difficult for others to keep up with their continuous flow of chatter as they pause to find the right words, and pick right up again. Not paying attention to them or not responding positively can cause disappointment and hurt feelings.

The Soulful diary is a great tool to encourage children to communicate their feelings positively in a confident compassionate way. It will help children identify and understand why and when they feel a certain way. Children will begin to take responsibility of their feelings and are given a safe place to express themselves freely.

Children can often go through a day of mixed emotions. Keeping a daily diary will help them decode their feelings, and constructively learn from all their experiences, the good, and the bad.

Adding gratitude to the diary helps maintain a positive approach to life, and helps children appreciate even the smallest of things and the role that others play in their lives. In the 21st century, the millennial children have far more possessions which go beyond their actual needs, such as expensive high-tech gadgets that even some adults do not possess. While technology is a must for our generation of children, they have lost the art of appreciation as they are given more things than they can use.

If taught properly, the gratitude diary will help your child be mindful of all the positivity in their lives, and they will have the opportunity to fully engage in and be grateful for anything they have been given. Adding gratitude is the best gift you can give your child. It's important to pay attention to both the emotional and physical well-being of your child.

Finally, positive affirmations are used to help children feel better, create positive attitudes, and achieve desired goals. These affirmations work better when positive emotions are internalized. When you affirm what you want, you mentally and emotionally make it true. I firmly believe in the concept of what we think we create.

Even one simple affirmation like "happiness surrounds me" has such a strong vibration. We have gone one step further and write the affirmations on our children's bedroom mirror. These affirmations can change as often as your child wants.

I am very passionate about this process, and I truly believe that by incorporating the daily diary writing into your child's life is one of the greatest gifts you can bestow upon them.

Soulful Diary questions & answers

My child is resisting the diary, what shall I do?

I would take a break and revisit it later. You can talk through the points as I think it's important to get them talking about gratitude, and the affirmations are powerful, too. Begin with saying them together.

Soulful Diaries

The following diaries are for older children; 9 onwards and younger children; from 3-8. You can find copies on my website, *www.essentialharmony.net*.

Daily Diary For Older Kids

Morning

Did you have a good night sleep?
Did you wake up by yourself or did someone wake you?

....

....

....

....

How do you feel this morning? Excited/happy/sad/tired…

....

....

....

....

Write down 1 or 2 goals you wish you could do today:

....

....

....

....

....

I love my family because:

....

....

....

....

Today I choose to be happy

I am full of light and love

I am positive and everything is possible

Before Bed

Describe how your day went. What was good and what could have been better?

....

....

....

Write down 2 things you are grateful for:

....

....

....

....

My loving thought before bed

....

....

....

....

....

All is well in my life.

I am special and full of love!

Daily Diary For Younger Kids

Did you Sleep well?

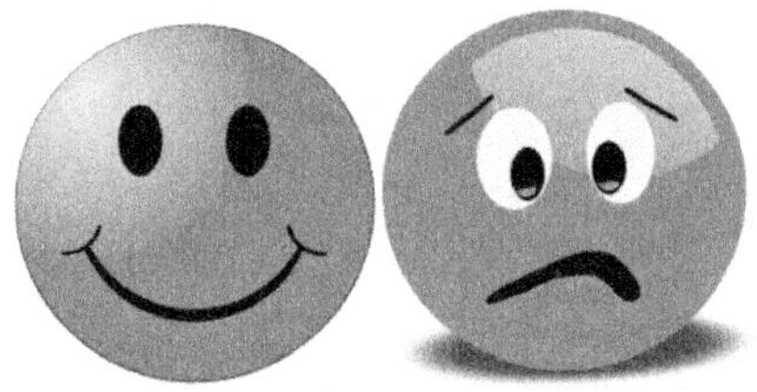

How do you feel this morning?

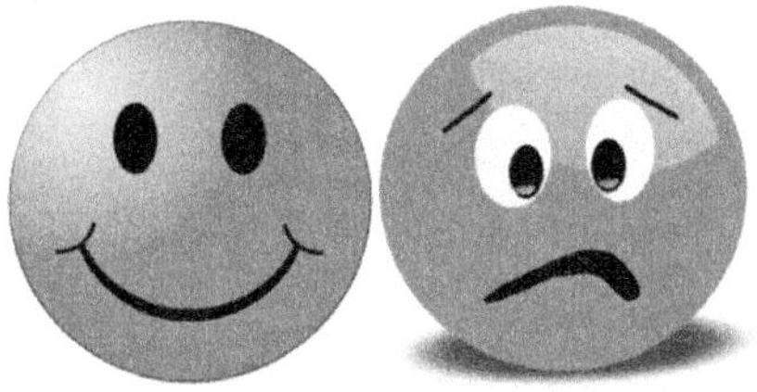

Say the following with your child:

Today I choose to be happy
I am full of light and love.
I am positive and everything is possible

Before Bed

How was your day?

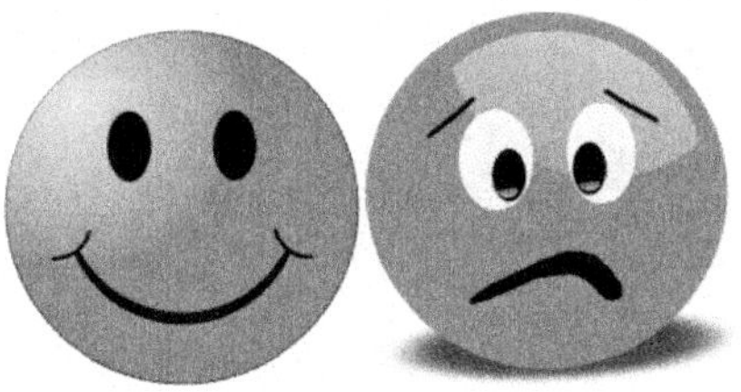

Did you eat a "Food Rainbow" today?

Color in the rainbow with the different fruits and vegetables you had.

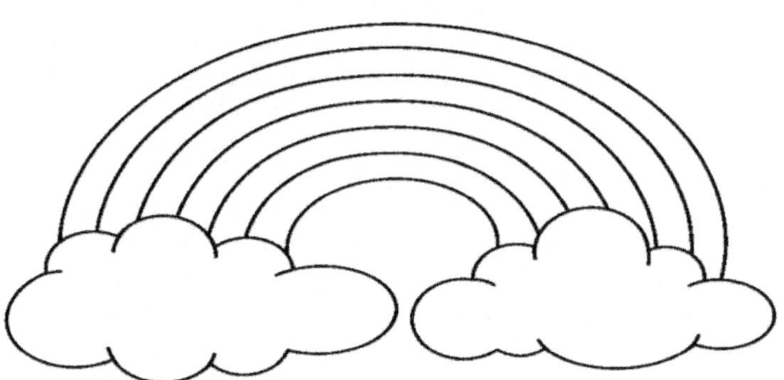

Tell your parent 2 things you are grateful for:

My loving thought before bed:

All is well in my life
I am special and full of love!

YOGA

Yoga is a form of exercise that is over 5,000 years old, and originates from India. It is an exercise for your mind, body and soul. The word "yoga" comes from the Sanskrit root 'yuj' which means "to unite." When your physical, intellectual, and spiritual selves are working in union, your life becomes balanced.

The practice of yoga enables you to achieve calmness, clarity, a sense of well-being, enthusiasm towards life, and peace of mind. Yoga is a powerful routine for enhancing your mind-body integration, which means you are establishing a healthy dialogue between your thoughts and your cells.

A yoga practice consists of various poses that are made up of breath work, stretching and relaxation. Each pose (asana) has its own unique benefit.

Therefore, combining various poses in a session will do wonders to your child. Yoga gives parents an alternative way to calm down children, and soothe their anxieties.

Benefits of children practicing yoga

- *Enhancing concentration:* Kids learn to sit still in one place and focuses on what is important during the session. After many sessions this can help them at school, boost their attention span, and potentially improve their grades.
- *Increasing flexibility and balance*: Through the different postures and asanas, your child will learn not just flexibility of the body, but of the mind, as well.
- *Improving general well-being*: Kids who practice yoga regularly feel good about themselves, become healthier and happier. After a few weeks, they may feel both mentally and physically rejuvenated after each session.
- *Boosts immunity:* Yoga's postures improve the flow of the lymphatic system, which is responsible for fighting infection and releasing toxins from the body.
- *Boosting confidence*: Kids get to develop their balance, strength, coordination, and flexibility through yoga. When children learn new skills, it boosts their confidence and independence.
- *Relaxing their minds*: Children are subject to a great deal of stress these days. They feel the need to be good at everything, and often feel very sad / stressed when they fail. Yoga gives children tools to help them relax more easily. It can help soothe their minds and ease away any worries that they may feel.

How to start a yoga session with your kids?

The following is an example of what my family does. You can adapt it to fit it into your own family life:

Yoga can be practiced any time of the day. Personally, we do it just before the children go to sleep. On the weekends, we may start the day off with a yoga session. You can also do it for 5 minutes or up to an hour. The key thing is to do it every day for as long as possible.

We practice yoga together in a room with minimal distractions. It's best to have a routine and try to stick to it. For example, tell the children that after brushing their teeth we will all meet in a room to do yoga. Children love structure.

The following pages contain various yoga poses, and easy-to-follow instructions.

Lotus Pose

First, make sure you "tune in" i.e step away from daily activities into yoga mode. Everyone sits in a circle, and in the lotus position and make sure the children sit tall. They can have the back of their hands on their knees with the thumb touching the forefinger or the hands together in prayer position against their heart. With eyes closed, you breath in (as tummy goes out) and then as you breath out (tummy goes in) you say "Om" the universal sound. 'Om' is a mantra often chanted during yoga classes for its vibrational quality. This sound will vibrate around the heart area. Repeat two more times.

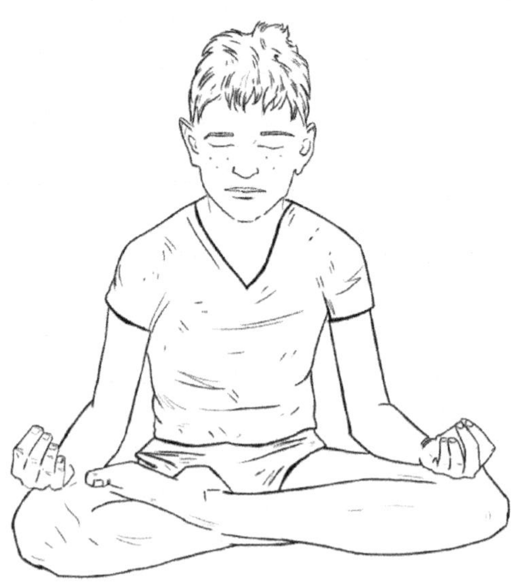

We then take turns and say, "*The light inside of me, shines the light inside of you*" When you say "*me*" point the hand towards yourself, and when you say "*you*" point it around your family. This sets the stage for sharing what we are grateful for. We each take turns saying what we are grateful for. It can be anything in general or about each other. If either of my two children are having a meltdown and being mean to each other, then I focus on saying something about each other that makes us grateful. This quick and simple technique gets them back to a happy and loving state.

We then go into the poses (asana). On a school night, we probably do between 4-6 poses and on the weekend/holidays we do around 8-10 different poses.

There are over 100 different poses to choose from. The following are the most popular poses in our household. Concentrate on a few and after you get comfortable with them, then you can explore other ones.

Mountain Pose

Mountain pose is the foundation for many of the standing yoga poses, therefore it is important to get it right. Like a mountain, your children can imagine standing tall and strong, and not falling when it is windy or stormy.

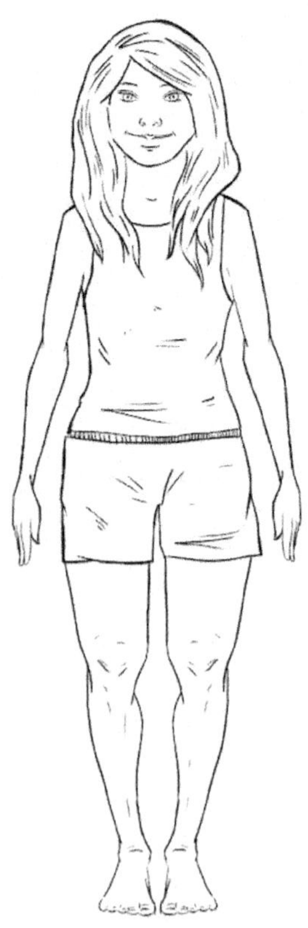

- Have your child stand tall with soft knees, focusing on a spot in front of them.
- Make sure their feet are facing forward and parallel, with the big toes touching.
- Have them firm their thigh muscles, lift their knees, pull in their belly, and stand tall.
- Their arms will hang on both sides of their tummy and their shoulders should be pulled back.
- While focusing on a spot in front of them, have them breathe deeply by inhaling and exhaling for about 1 minute.

The Mountain Pose cultivates strength, improved posture, concentration and calmness.

Tree Pose

Like a tree, your children can stand tall and imagine roots growing from their feet into the ground. You can either spread out the arms like branches to accept the light and love from the sun and energy from the roots to the finger tips, or you can put the hands to your heart like below. This pose is grounding and connects us to mother earth.

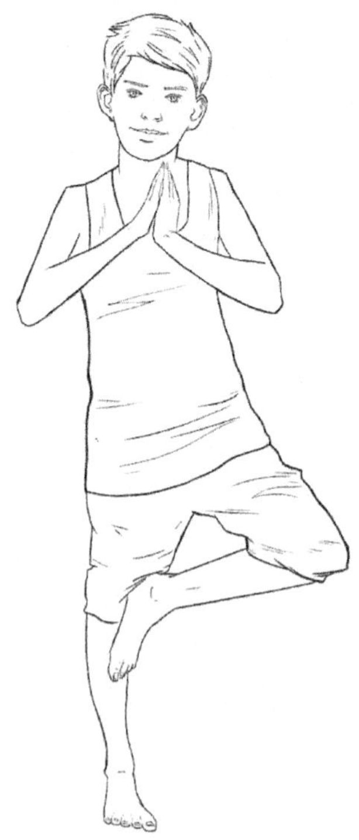

- Start with a mountain pose and stand strong.
- While one foot is pressed firmly on the ground, the opposite foot is raised to rest on the standing leg, above or just below the knee.
- Bring the arm to the chest in a praying position. Hold this position for as long as possible.
- If you want to take it further, raise the arms and stretch them out wide like limbs of a tree. Then spread out the finger branches.
- Hold the position for as long as possible, and then switch sides.

I get my daughter to focus on my finger, this seems to help her hold the pose longer.

The Tree Pose improves balance, concentration and focus. If you have more than one child, you can hold hands and form a forest.

Warrior Pose

Like a warrior, you need to stand strong and ready for attack. In yoga, the “attack” is representative of life’s ups and down, and the warrior stands strong and handles each obstacle peacefully. Children are faced with so many stresses with school work, activities and home life. This pose will help you feel strong within, and without hurting anyone.

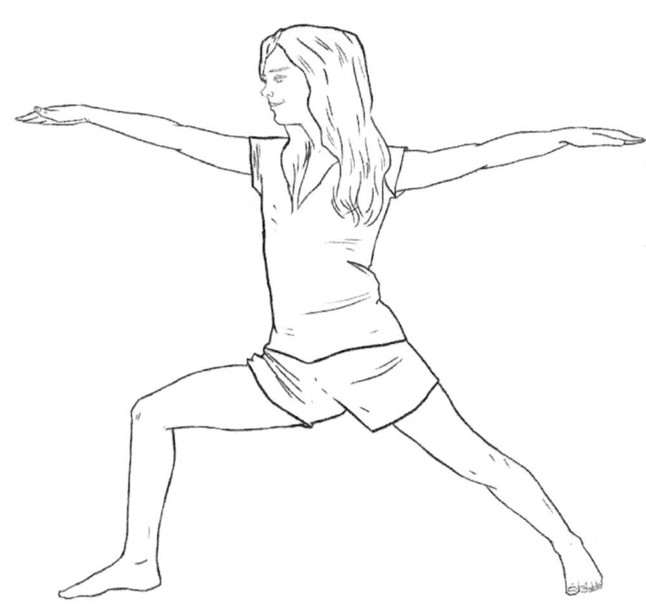

- Stand strong with both feet pointing forward and legs width apart.
- Turn your left foot in, and right foot forward. Back is straight.
- Stretch your hands, and raise them up to your shoulders.
- Look towards the fingertips of the right hand.
- Stay in this position for a few seconds.
- Lower your hands, and straighten your legs while inhaling.
- Repeat this pose on the other side.

The warrior pose strengthens the legs and opens the chest. It builds stamina, and improves balance and confidence.

Cat and Cow Pose

These two poses can be done separately but doing them together helps stretch out the back more efficiently. We love this pose! Like a cat stretches his back looking upwards, this is what happens in the cat pose. The cow pose in the inverted stretch while looking downwards. Together they help stretch out your child's back especially after a long day at school slumped in front of their desk.

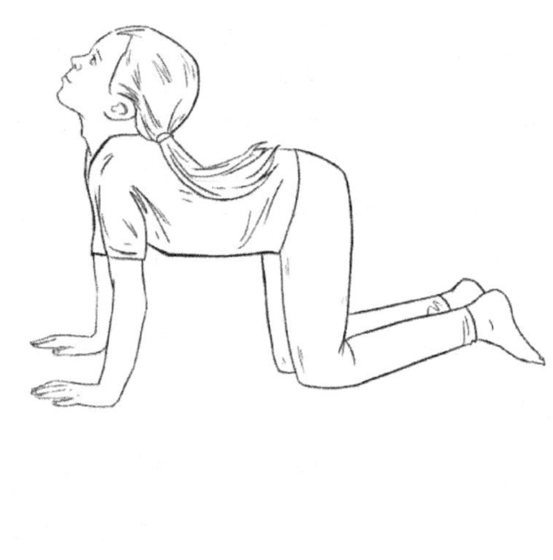

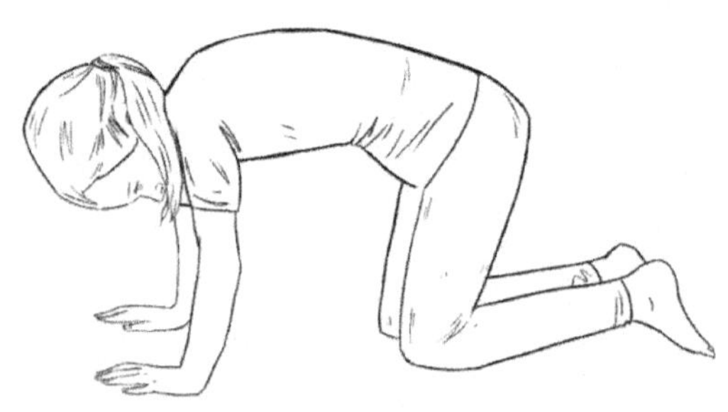

- Kneel down with your knees underneath your hips and hands should be underneath your shoulders.
- Hands should be straight and elbows should not be bent.
- Let your tummy slightly sink towards the floor while inhaling. Look towards the ceiling. (Cat pose)
- Now, exhale and slightly raise your tummy towards the ceiling. Look towards your belly. (Cow pose)
- Repeat this pose 2-3 times. Make sure these two poses are done nice and slowly so the back can be fully stretched out.

The cow/cat pose helps stretch the neck and spinal cord. It also massages the organs. These two poses together helps your child understand about fluidity and flow.

Downward Dog Pose

This pose is one of the most popular amongst children and it is easy to grasp. The hands and feet act like the four paws of a dog. The downward dog pose emphasizes stretching and strengthening the spine.

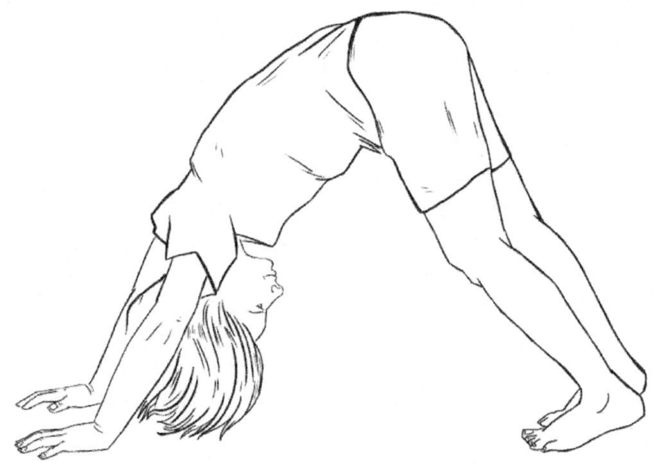

- Start out on all fours like a table.
- Spread your fingers and press your palms flat onto the floor.
- Lift your bottom, straighten your legs, and make an upside-down V shape.
- Send your heels gently to the ground.
- Relax your head and neck, and look down between your legs.

The downward dog pose has many benefits but the main ones are that it eliminates stiffness in the back, especially after a long day at school sitting in a chair. It also boosts circulation which helps flush out toxins and boost the immune system.

Lying Down Spinal Twist pose

This is my favorite pose as it helps stretch my back and wrings out all the tension and tightness I experience after standing or sitting for long periods. My children love this pose for the same reason.

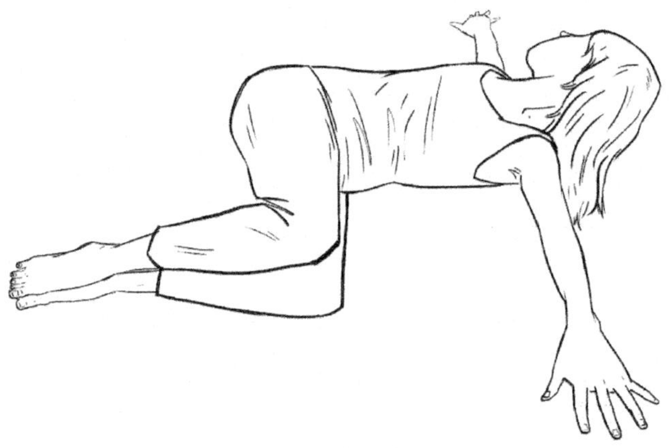

- Lie on your back.
- Hug your knees and roll left to right, gently massaging the back. Return to the centre.
- While legs are straight, stretch the arms out by your shoulders with the palm facing up. You should look like a cross.
- Inhale and bend your knee and hips to the right side, and your ribs, neck and head to the the left side. Arms are still straight. Exhale. Hold for about a minute.
- Change sides and repeat 5 times.

Once finished, release to the right side and relax. Breathe in and out deeply and close your eyes to help further relax.

This pose nourishes the spine, body and organs. It massages, strengthens and encourages the blood flow.

Child Pose

This is the first pose many children are taught. It's simple to do and has great benefits. It's a great stretching and relaxing pose. We normally do the child pose in-between a couple of other poses. It helps relax the body, especially if you have been holding a pose for a long time.

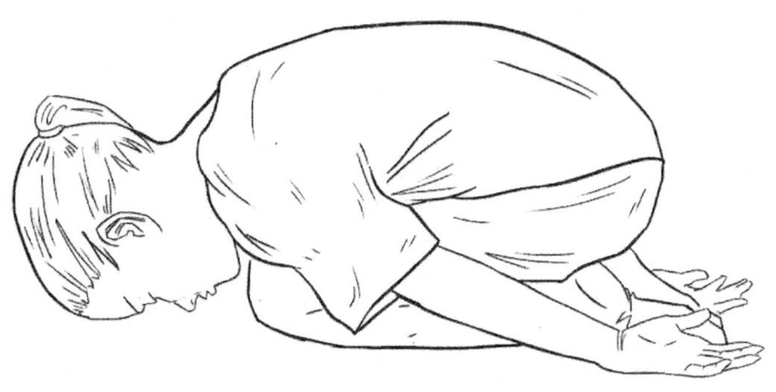

- Sit on your knees with your feet together and your bottom on your heels. Get comfortable.
- Inhale deeply and as you exhale bring your chest down over your thighs. The arms will be forward with the palms of your hands facing down.
- While resting with your forehead on the ground bring your arms around your sides and rest your hands palms facing up.
- As a rock, relax and stay still for about 1 minute.

The child pose not only offers the child a gentle stretch of the back, knees, ankles and thighs, it also helps the child connect with mother earth and brings peace and harmony to the child's body.

Cobra Pose

While children are at their desks all day, they tend to slump their shoulders forward. As the cobra pose is a heart opener pose, it is a great remedy for the bad effects caused by slouching.

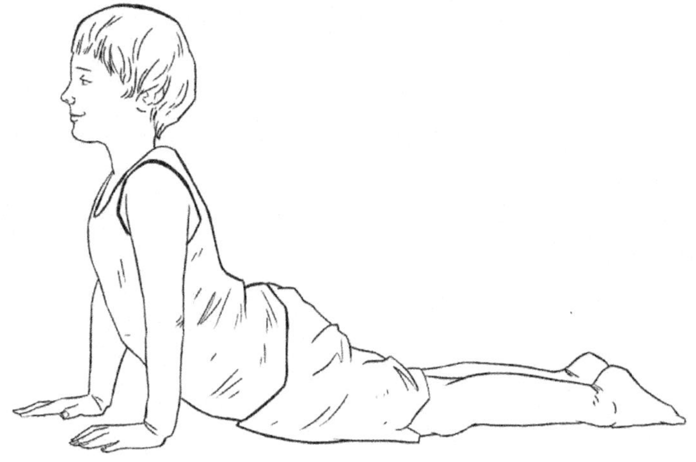

- Begin on your belly with your legs together and place your palms face-down underneath your head.
- Raise your head and place your hands underneath your shoulders.
- Raise further up and press on your hands while you arch up.
- Keep raising and while the chest is opening, the arms are almost straight.

The cobra pose has many benefits. While you are

opening the heart area and chest, you are also strengthening the lungs and this is a great pose during the cold/flu season. It massages the abdomen and aides digestion.

Yoga questions & answers

My two children laugh through the session and I get frustrated.

If you set the scene and maybe dim the lights and play soft music, this will help calm them down. I would start it off with three deep breaths and this will centre them.

My kids don't get the poses right.

That is perfectly fine, it takes time and practice. They will soon be professional yoga students.

My daughter likes some of the poses and she doesn't want to do the others.

That is perfectly fine also. The purpose of yoga for kids is to help calm them down. If she doesn't want to do a certain pose, try another one.

MEDITATION

Meditation has different meanings to different people. Some people feel that meditation helps them with relaxation and stress management. Other people may find that meditation helps them go deeper in their being and soul to connect to the higher self whether that is God, the angels or spirit. For me, it helps me connect to the present time, and value what is going on NOW in my life; not the future or past.

I believe that we owe it to our children to introduce meditation into their lives from a young age. I see many adults who have taken on meditation after an illness, stress at work, or even a divorce. It helps them bring some "calm" back to their lives after the "storm."

Life for a child in the 21st century can be stressful. They are pulled in so many directions whether it is school work, sports, friends, or music. Meditation is a powerful tool that helps your child breathe and stay focused on the here and now. This will hopefully, in time, give them the skills to be mindful of their day instead of each day mixing in with the next and they lose the joy of their childhood! Meditation can also help your child diffuse any negativity or drama that they may be experiencing.

I introduced meditation into my children's lives two years ago. You can literally see their anxieties melt away and their breathing slow down. It is a seed that is planted within them that they can call upon anytime in their life. As they see and witness the benefit that meditation has on me, they do not question it. Recently, we all took part in a global meditation, and it was a blessing to see my children sit and breath softly for over 10 minutes. They awoke much calmer and they had a glow to their aura.

Meditation normally follows a yoga session. Your children are already nice and calm, and any aches and pains have been eased away. You can add to the calmed setting by dimming the lights and infusing essentials oils, for example lavender.

Meditation for children can be anything from lying down and you reading a calming story to sitting in a lotus position and they repeat a mantra over and over again softly or in their mind for about five minutes.

If your child is not happy with the concept of meditation, then you can call it a concentration practice.

The beauty of meditation is that you can focus on anything and change it to what is relevant to your family. For example, if your child is anxious about his/her first day at school, then you could sit in a lotus position and ask them to repeat, "All will be well" over and over until you can see him relaxing and calming down.

Another option is that they lie down and close

their eyes while they listen to you read a "calming" story. I sometimes make up a story and base it around a holiday destination where I take them on an adventure with me.

Once you get your child interested in meditation and they start noticing the benefits, all else will fall into place. Your children have been given a precious gift that they can use for the rest of their lives.

Some examples

Breathing techniques: First, breathe in with the count to three, hold and then breathe out with the count of three. As you breathe in, you breathe in love, peace and energy. As you hold, these feelings are spreading around the body. As you breathe out, imagine any sadness, anger and frustration leaving your body.

Focusing techniques: As they lie down or sit in a lotus position, your child will concentrate on a mantra. They will repeat it slowly first by saying it, then whisper it, and then finally silently in their mind. There are several mantras out there but we like "peace within me."

Speaking meditation: This is when you guide them along a journey. Make sure that the tone of your voice is calm, slow and relaxed. When saying the meditation, pause for reflection, and keep it slow. This will help your child focus on the words that you are saying, and they will remain relaxed.

A column of white light

"A beautiful column of bright light is flowing down on you. It flows down on your head, helping your head relax.

You feel your head relaxing. It moves down over your face, through your neck and around your shoulders. Your face, neck and shoulders are relaxing.

The bright light flows down through your arms to your fingers. You feel your arms and fingers relaxing. It flows down your back, and you begin to relax and release any tension.

It flows over your chest and your stomach. You are nice and relaxed.

It moves down over your legs and feet. You feel your legs and feet letting go and relaxing.

The beautiful white light is shining over your entire body.

As you breathe in and out, the white light gets stronger and stronger.

You are surrounded by love and peace. You are very peaceful and relaxed."

Rainbow Meditation

"Imagine your body as a white light. Breathe in and out this bright light.

Now imagine a rainbow in the sky. The rainbow is shining with all the colors, and each color will pour into you. Slowly, you become the red color. You are strong and energized with the red. Feel the red all around your body. Breathe it in and out.

Now watch the bright orange enter your body. Slowly you become the orange color. You are grounded with happiness and joy. Feel the orange all around your body. Breathe it in and out. Now watch the bright yellow enter your body.

Slowly, you become the yellow color. You are warm and powerful. Feel the yellow all around your body. Breathe it in and out. Now, watch the green color enter your body. Slowly, you become the green color. You are loved and nurtured. Feel the green all around your body. Breathe it in and out.

Now, watch the blue color enter your body. Slowly, you become the blue color. You can communicate all you wish for. Feel the blue all around your body. Breathe it in and out. Now, watch the indigo color enter your body. Slowly, you become the indigo color. You are wise and thoughtful. Feel the indigo all around your body. Breathe it in and out. Now, watch the bright violet color enter your body.

Slowly, you become the violet color. You are love. Feel the violet all around your body. Breathe it in and out. You are the rainbow full of all these colors. Where ever you go, you are full of brightness. The colors are in your heart, and you are now this beautiful shining rainbow inside and out."

Meditation Questions & Answers

My child just falls asleep during meditation?

That is perfectly fine. What I suggest is after yoga, take the meditation to their room and let your child lie down in bed. This is a perfect way to fall asleep.

Is it better for my child to sit cross-legged during meditation or lying down?

When children start meditating, I recommend them to lie down as sitting often causes them to fidget. Once they are comfortable with the concept of meditation, then I would try to get them to sit in a lotus position. They may only last a few minutes, so start off small.

PART IV
HEALTHY MEALS TO ENJOY

BREAKFAST

Starting the day off with a good hearty breakfast will help keep your children's blood sugar stable. The brain needs various nutrients to help it function, therefore taking time and effort to ensure that your children start the day off on the right foot will be beneficial to everyone.

Most children I know start the day off with a bowl of cereal, which in most cases are loaded with sugar, and are limited in nutritional value. They are not filling, and your child is more likely to be hungry in no time.

Ensuring that your children have some complex carbohydrates and/or protein will not only help stabilize their blood sugar, but they will be satisfied for much longer.

The breakfast ideas I have included are easy to prepare. Try them to see which ones are a hit with your children. There are plenty more options out there. If your child prefers the smoothie, then you can experiment by adding nuts, seeds, or even quinoa flakes. Adding nutritional value to their breakfast is key. Another option, which I have not included, is toast. Choose whole wheat (please check the ingredients for any additives). On the toast, you can add nut butters, eggs, avocado, smoked salmon, or you can even add baked beans. This simple breakfast is quick and easy, and will give your children a healthy start to the day.

Almond Pancakes

Makes 4 servings ***Prep:*** *10 minutes,* ***Cooking:*** *10 minutes*

1 egg,

1 ½ cups almond milk

¼ cup of extra light Olive oil

1 ¾ cups oat or whole wheat pastry flour

½ cup almonds, finely chopped

1 tbsp non-aluminum baking powder

½ tsp sea salt

- Mix egg, milk and oil in a medium-size bowl.
- Mix flour, almonds, baking powder and salt into a small bowl.
- Combine dry ingredients into the wet ingredients.
- Mix until dry ingredients are moistened.
- Using a 1/4…1/2 cup measuring cup drop pancakes onto a lightly oiled skillet and cook until golden brown on both sides.
- Serve warm with maple syrup or honey

Try a little lemon zest, the juice of one lemon (add a little less milk) and 1/2 cup poppy seeds for lemon poppy seed pancakes.

Easy Flour free Banana Pancakes

Makes 2 servings, ***Prep:*** *2 minutes,* ***Cooking:*** *5 minutes*

1 ripe banana, mashed
2 eggs
Coconut oil for frying

- Whisk the eggs in a bowl
- Mix in the banana
- Put your skillet/frying pan on a medium-low heat and add 1tbsp coconut oil
- Cook until golden brown on both sides (1-2 minutes on each side).
- Top with fresh berries

Seyan's wake me up Smoothie

Makes 2 servings, ***Prep:*** *2 minutes*

2 banana
15 strawberries
2 table spoons coconut milk
¼ cup ice cubes

- Place in a blender on high
- Serve in a tall glass

Chai seed delight

Makes 2 servings, ***Prep time:*** *Overnight, next day 2 Minutes*

2 tbsp. chia seeds

½ cup almond milk

Honey to sweeten

Mixed berries/fruit e.g sliced strawberries , sliced bananas...

- Soak the chia seeds in the almond milk overnight.

The next day top with the fruit and add honey to sweeten

Easy Homemade Granola

Makes 3 servings, ***Prep:*** *5 minutes,* ***Cooking:*** *15 minutes*

2 cups rolled oats

½ cup slivered almonds

½ cup dried shredded coconut

¼ cup crystallized ginger, chopped into smaller pieces

¼ cup coconut oil

¼ cup maple syrup

- Preheat oven to 350 F.
- Combine all ingredients into a large bowl.
- Spread in a thin layer on a cookie sheet.
- Bake for 5 minutes and then stir with a spatula and spread evenly.
- Bake another 5 minutes stir/spread again.
- Finally, bake for 15 minutes until golden brown all over.
- Cool for about 10 minutes prior to serving
- Can be stored for up to a week in an air tight container, best stored at room temperature.

Oatmeal Pancakes or Waffles

Makes 2 servings, ***Prep:*** *10 minutes,* ***Cooking:*** *10 minutes*

2 cups rolled oats

2 cups water

1 banana

2 tbsp maple syrup

¼ tsp sea salt

1 tsp vanilla extract

Extra light olive oil or coconut oil for frying/waffle iron

- Place all ingredients, except oil, in a blender and blend until smooth.
- Stand a few minutes until batter thickens.
- If too thick to pour easily, add some water.
- Heat oil in frying pan or skillet.
- *Pancakes:* Pour batter (¼~½ cup) into pan and cook for 2-3 minutes on each side.
- *Waffles:* lightly brush waffle iron with oil, pour mixture into the heated waffle iron and cook for 10 minutes.

Olivia's Yummy Porridge

Two servings, ***Prep:*** *Soak oats overnight,* ***Cooking:*** *6 mins*

½ cup Rolled Oats

1 tsp almond butter

½ tsp cinnamon

1 cup almond milk

- Put oats and half the milk into a saucepan
- Bring to the boil then turn down to simmer for 4-5 minutes
- As it thickens stir in the remaining milk
- Add the almond butter, mashing it into the porridge
- Dish porridge into two bowls
- Sprinkle the cinnamon on top

Scrambled eggs Nishma Style!

*Makes 2 servings, **Prep:** 2 minutes, **Cooking:** 6 minutes*

3 eggs

2 tbsp cilantros

½ tsp of turmeric

Pinch of red chili powder

3 tbsp of cold water

2 tsp of coconut oil or butter for frying

- Whisk all ingredients together until light and foamy
- Put a frying pan on medium-high heat and add butter/coconut oil
- Once melted add egg mixture to the pan
- Stir eggs slowly, as soon as it starts to thicken reduce the heat and bring thick parts of the mixture into the middle.
- Once cooked turn it out on to the warmed plate.

Scrambled eggs can lose their heat very quickly so avoid putting them straight onto a cold plate, either warm the plates in the oven or in hot water in the sink.

LUNCH & DINNER

Lunch

In my opinion, most school lunches in the United States need a lot of improvement. If your child is having a school lunch, please look into what is being offered, and have a look at the ingredients that are used to make the meals. Ensure that these meals are providing your child with the nutrients required to live a healthy life.

If you decide to send a packed lunch, there are many healthy options out there.

With sandwiches, there are many varieties of bread available, and there are many different fillings to try. With bread, if we make it from scratch, we normally use flour, water, salt and yeast. When we go to the supermarket, there are so many varieties, and some that I have seen have over 15 ingredients. So, please be mindful of the bread you choose, and what it contains.

You can try many fillings, from cheese, tuna, egg, hummus, peanut butter, chicken, salad, and so forth. It is important to include protein because it helps stabilize the bloods sugar, and it will satisfy your child for a longer period of time.

Salads are another healthy option. This may be a better choice for the older children. Along with the salad leaves, include various vegetables, such as peppers, cucumber, broccoli or even mushrooms. You can add chicken, tuna, beans, lentils, hummus, or eggs to add much needed protein to the salad.

Finally, you can send a hot meal. This could be soup, meat with rice, beans with rice, or even pasta. You can get a thermos, which is great for children's lunch boxes.

As you can see, there are many options to choose from when we are considering children's lunches, and most of these do not take much time to prepare. The main point to remember is that what you feed your children on a regular basis will affect their well-being over time, so make the choices optimal.

Dinner

This meal can be tricky. With so many after-school activities, sometimes the easy option is take-out or a processed meal. I have included some meals, which do take time to cook, but they are full of a lot of nutrients that will benefit your child.

With some of the meals, you can batch cook them and freeze for another day to enjoy. We prepare several meals over the weekend and freeze them, so when time is not on our side, we can at least guarantee that the children are eating healthy those days too.

Noodles with tofu

Makes 4 servings, ***Prep:*** *20 minutes,* ***Cooking:*** *40 minutes*

250g (approx) block of Tofu

1 Red onion peeled and thinly sliced

1 tsp ginger finely chopped/minced

2 cloves of garlic, crushed

1 large or 2 small bell peppers (red/yellow/orange) deseeded and thinly sliced

1 Zucchini peeled and thinly sliced

1 cup broccoli chopped into small flowerets

1 tbsp of dark (or 2 of light) soy sauce

1 tbsp of extra light Olive oil

Dried Noodles

Baking (greaseproof) paper

- Preheat the oven to 350 F
- Drain the tofu and remove excess liquid by wrapping it in paper towel and gently squeezing it, be careful not to tear the tofu
- Slice the tofu into 5mm thick rectangles, place onto baking paper on a baking tray and put in the oven for 10 minutes
- Put the oil in a wok or large frying pan, over a medium-high heat
- Once hot add onions and cook for a minute
- Add garlic, ginger, peppers, Zucchini cook for 2 minutes and take off the heat
- Once the 10 minutes is up for the tofu, turn each piece over and put it back in the oven for another 10 minutes
- When the tofu is nearly done, put the dried noodles in a saucepan and cover with boiling water
- Put the wok back on a medium heat, sprinkle sugar, stir and cook for a minute then add soy sauce and cook for a further minute
- Drain the noodles then mix with the tofu mixture while still in the wok, serve.

David's Delicious Quiches

Makes ~ 16 quiches, ***Prep:*** *40 mins,* ***Cooking:*** *30-40 mins*

For the short crust (pie) pastry

125g Plain Flour

125g Whole wheat Flour

110g Butter

60-90 ml ice cold water

For filling

1 tbsp of extra light Olive oil

1 Onion peeled and finely chopped

1 clove of garlic, crushed

½ cup corn kernels

1 cup broccoli chopped into small flowerets

1 Bell Pepper deseeded and chopped into small pieces

100g of grated cheddar cheese

250 ml (1 cup) milk

2 eggs

1 tsp mixed herbs

12 hole muffin tin
Rub butter into each pan (each pan approximately 7cm (2 ¾") across)

Pastry cutter ~8.5 cm (3 ½")

- Shift flours together
- Cut butter into small cubes, add to flour
- Using your fingertips rub the butter into the flour until it resembles breadcrumbs
- Gradually add the ice cold water stirring it with a table knife
- Tip mixture on to a floured surface and gently knead into a ball
- Cover with cling film and pop in the fridge for at least 15 minutes.
- Preheat the oven to 400 F
- Put oil in a large frying pan, over a medium-high heat
- Once hot add onions, cook for a minute
- Add garlic, peppers, corn, broccoli, herbs and salt/pepper to taste
- Cook stirring occasionally until done (approx 6 mins). Once done take off heat
- Whisk eggs, milk in a jug for easy pouring
- Take out pastry and roll on a floured surface until approximately 5mm thick.
- Cut pastry and gently press/stretch each pastry circle into each pan
- Mix grated cheese into the filling then put a teaspoon of filling into each quiche case.
- Pour the egg mixture into each quiche case, filling it about two-thirds.
- Bake for 20 minutes, the quiches should be brown on top with no runny egg.

Conor's Hidden Veggies Red Sauce

This tomato based sauce is a great way of getting kids to eat more vegetables without them even realizing it. Once made it can be frozen and used as a base for Nachos, pasta, pizza, Shepard's pie...

Makes 4 servings, ***Prep:*** *15 minutes,* ***Cooking:*** *40 minutes*

- **1 tbsp of extra light Olive oil**
- **1 Onion peeled and finely chopped**
- **2 Cloves of garlic, crushed**
- **2 Small or one large leek sliced**
- **1 Carrot peeled and chopped**
- **1 Zucchini peeled and thinly sliced**
- **1 Bell pepper deseeded and chopped**
- **60 g of split red lentils washed and soaked**
- **1 1/2 tsp of mixed herbs**
- **1 tsp of sugar**
- **2 tins of chopped tomatoes (~400g each)**
- **1 veggie stock cube and 400 ml of boiling water OR 400 ml of veggie stock**

Put the stock cube in a jug and then pour over the boiling water

Put the oil in a large sauce pan, over a medium heat

Once hot add onions and cook for a minute

Add the remaining vegetables (garlic, leeks, pepper, carrot, zucchini) and cook for another 3-5 minutes, stirring occasionally

Add the vegetable stock and turn down to a simmer

Drain and add the lentils

Add both tins of chopped tomatoes

Add the mixed herbs

Let it simmer for 20-30 minutes, stirring occasionally, until the lentils are soft to touch

Once cooled use a hand blender or kitchen whiz to process it to a smooth puree consistency

Cheese Sauce

Base sauce for a dish for 4, ***Cooking****: 15 minutes*

This is a very versatile sauce that can be used as a base of a lot of dishes (lasagna, Mac Cheese, Cauliflower/Broccoli bake...). The secret is to add hot milk which makes it easier to cook and produces a creamer sauce.

4 tbsp butter

1 ½ cups of milk

3 tbsp flour

2 gloves of garlic, crushed

¾ cup of grated cheese

Ground pepper

- Heat milk with a sprinkle of pepper to boiling point then take off heat
- Melt butter in a new saucepan, and add garlic, cook for a minute
- Take butter off heat, add flour and stir in well
- Slowly add the hot milk, stirring
- Once you've added about two thirds of the milk put in back on a medium heat and stir until it becomes very thick. Back off the heat and slowly add the remaining milk, stirring.
- Add half the cheese and return sauce to a medium heat to melt it

NikNok's Creamy Lasagna

Makes 4 serving, ***Prep****:20 minutes,* ***Cooking****: 1 hour*

For best results cook the lasagna the day before, that way you get a nice firm lasagna that sits much better on your plate.

I also prefer to boil the lasagna even if it is "oven ready"

15 Sheets of dried Lasagna (~400g)

2 cups Hidden Veggies Red Sauce (see above)

Cheese sauce (see above)

2 tbsp of extra light Olive oil

300g mushrooms washed and sliced

1 large Onion peeled and sliced

2 Zucchinis peeled and sliced

1 red/yellow bell pepper deseeded and sliced

1 cup of grated cheese

Ground pepper

- Pre-heat the oven to 400F
- Bring a large saucepan of water to the boil add a tbsp of oil
- Cook the lasagna sheets for about 6 minutes, do a few sheets at a time so they don't stick together
- Heat oil in a frying pan over a medium heat
- Add onions and cook for a minute
- Add bell pepper, zucchini, stir and cook for 2 minutes
- Add mushrooms, stir and cook for a final 2 minutes
- Spread a little red sauce on the bottom of a lasagna dish, place a layer of lasagna sheets on this
- Spread over a third of the red sauce, half the veggies and a third of the cheese sauce
- Cover with a layer of pasta sheets and repeat.
- On the top layer put the remaining cheese sauce and sprinkle grated cheese over the top
- Bake for 20-30 minutes until golden brown

Izzy's Pasta Bake

Makes 4 servings, Prep: 15 mins, Cooking: 30 mins

Cheese sauce (see above)

A large head of Broccoli chopped into florets

A large head of Cauliflower chopped in florets

300g of macaroni pasta shells

1 cup of grated cheese

- Preheat the oven 400F
- Boil Broccoli and Cauliflower for 10 mins
- Bring a large pot of water to a boil over medium heat. Salt the water and add the broccoli and cauliflower florets. Boil the vegetables for 8 minutes, then remove them and strain
- Boil the pasta for 10 minutes (or as per cooking instructions.
- Once done drain the pasta and add the cooked vegetables.
- Stir through the cheese sauce, then transfer into a baking dish
- Sprinkle cheese over the top and put in the oven for 20 minutes until golden brown. As everything is precooked, if it's not quite golden switch to a low grill for a couple of minutes.

Sami's Tacos/ Tortilla Wraps

Makes 4 servings, ***Prep:*** *15 minutes,* ***Cooking:*** *20 minutes*

Bean Mixture

10-12 Corn Tacos or Tortillas

2 tins of Red kidney beans washed and drained

1 onion finely chopped

***1 tsp Cumin powder**

***½ tsp chili powder**

½ cup Hidden Veggies Red Sauce (see above)

1 tbsp of extra light Olive oil

Guacamole

2 ripe avocadoes

1 garlic glove crushed

2 tbsp fresh lime/lemon juice

¼ cup finely chopped red onions

2 tbsp cilantro finely chopped

Ground black pepper

Pinch of salt

Fillings

Iceberg lettuce washed, sliced

Tomatoes washed and cut into small cubes

Grated cucumber & carrot

Grated cheese

Greek yoghurt or soured cream as preferred

- Preheat the oven to 400F (for the Tacos)
- Coarsely mash the kidney beans
- Heat the oil in a frying pan on a medium heat
- Add onions and cook for a minute
- Add spices, stir, then add the kidney beans and stir until combined
- Sir in the red sauce, then reduce the heat to a low simmer, cook for a few minutes and take off the heat
- Put the avocadoes in a bowl and mash
- Add onions, garlic, and lemon juice to avocadoes and mix in
- Add black pepper and cilantro and carefully stir in
- Place tacos upside down on an oven tray and in the oven for a few minutes or if you're having wraps then warm up wraps
- Reheat the bean mixture
- Serve everything to the table, to make tacos put a little cheese in the bottom, spread the bean mixture on one side, add lettuce, tomatoes, cucumber, carrots and then a little guacamole and yoghurt on top
- We find letting the children put their own tacos together adds to the experience and means they're more likely to eat more.

** If your children don't like spicy food then leave out the spices*

Nehal's tasty Pesto Pasta

Makes 4 servings, ***Prep:*** *15 minutes,* ***Cooking:*** *30 minutes*

3 cups packed fresh Basil leaves washed and drained

½ cup roasted pine nuts

Juice of a lemon

2 cloves of garlic

¼ cup extra virgin olive oil

5 medium-large sized potatoes peeled, cubed and cover in hot salted water

2-3 tbsp extra light Olive oil for roasting potatoes

Ground black pepper

1 tsp dried rosemary

300g spaghetti or linguine pasta

⅓ cup grated Parmesan cheese or cheddar cheese as preferred

- Preheat the oven to 400F
- Add oil to a roasting pan, sprinkle black pepper and rosemary
- Place the pan in the oven for 5 minutes
- Drain the potatoes, making sure they're well drained
- Carefully add the potatoes to the roasting pan, sake or stir to finely cover in the oil, pepper and rosemary
- Place potatoes in the oven and cook for 20 minutes
- Add the basil, pine nuts, garlic in a blender/food processor and blend until everything is finely chopped
- Add the lemon juice and extra virgin olive oil to the basil and process for another minute until finely mixed
- Two-thirds fill a large sauce pan with water and bring to the boil
- Add the pasta and stir to stop it sticking
- Cook the pasta for 10 minutes (or as per instructions on the pack)
- Check potatoes, if not ready then turn them over and cook further
- Once the pasta is ready, drain, then return to the saucepan and add the pesto (enough as is needed to cover)
- Add the roast potatoes to the pasta and gently stir in
- Finally add the cheese, stir in and serve.

Healthy Cauliflower Pizza

Makes 1 large pizza, ***Prep:*** *15 minutes,* ***Cooking:*** *30 minutes*

Pizza Crust

1/2 head cauliflower

2 tbsp almond meal (ground almonds)

1 tsp oregano

1 egg

1/2 cup Hidden Veges Red Sauce (see above)

Grated Cheese

Topping ideas

Mushrooms, bell peppers chopped, corn kernels, red onion finely chopped

Roast potatoes and squash, rosemary, red onion finely sliced, goat's cheese

Kale or spinach leaves, raisins, red onion finely chopped, an egg cracked over the center

- Pre heat the oven to 350F
- Put the chopped cauliflower in a food processor or blender until it's fine
- Add to a bowl, cover and microwave on high for 5 minutes (or cover with boiling water and put over a medium heat for 5).
- Pour over a clean kitchen towel and allow to cool, then squeeze out all excess liquid. The more liquid you get out the better it will stay together when cooked.
- Add the rest of your ingredients into a bowl with the cauliflower and mix with your hands until well combined.
- On a cookie sheet lined with parchment paper, spread your mixture to roughly 2cm thick.
- Bake for 20 minutes or until it's lightly browned.
- Take out of the oven and spoon over the red sauce, spread evenly with the back of a spoon
- Add your toppings
- cover with grated cheese
- bake in the oven for 15 minutes or until golden brown

Nani's special Pudla (Indian Savory pancakes)

Makes 8-10 pancakes, ***Prep:*** *15 mins,* ***Cooking:*** *30 mins*

1 ½ cups of broccoli finely chopped

1 carrot grated

2 cups of gram flour

1 tsp of Turmeric

1 tsp of salt

1 ½ tsp of sugar

½ cup of cilantro, finely chopped

[Optional] 1 small green chili, remove seeds, finely chopped

2 cups of cold water

Extra light Olive oil or Coconut oil for frying

- Pour boiling water over the broccoli. Cover and leave to sit for 5 minutes
- Combine the dry ingredients into a large mixing bowl
- Make a well in the center and slowly add the water whilst stirring, if mixture is too thick add more water. It should be runny, the consistency of single cream
- If broccoli are soft then drain and mash with a potato masher if not boil for a couple of minutes then mash
- Add the mashed veggies and grated carrots to the mixture and stir well
- Lastly add cilantro and stir gently, once combined cover and leave to sit for 15 minutes
- Drizzle a tsp of oil in non-stick frying pan over a hot heat,
- Reduce the heat to medium high and pour a ¼ - ½ cup of mixture into the frying pan, then spread evenly using the back of a spoon
- Cook for about 30 seconds (until brown) then turn over carefully, you may need to loosen the edges
- Cook for another 30 seconds or until brown

Kian's Black Bean Veggie Burger

Makes 6-8 pancakes, ***Prep:*** *20 minutes,* ***Cooking:*** *15 minutes*

Bean Patties

400 g (15 oz) tin of black beans washed and drained

1 onion finely chopped

1 clove of garlic crushed

1 tsp of cumin

1 tsp of ground coriander

Some ground pepper to taste

Plain flour for making into patties

Extra light Olive oil or Coconut oil for frying

Burger Filling

Pack of burger buns or soft rolls

Cheddar cheese sliced

Iceberg lettuce leaves

Cucumber sliced

Sliced red onion

Tomato sliced

Tomato sauce and Mayonnaise

- Mash the black beans using a potato masher
- Heat a table spoon of oil in a frying pan over a medium heat
- Add onion and cook for a couple of minutes
- Add garlic, cumin and coriander and cook for a further minute
- Add onion/spice mixture to the mashed beans and stir in well
- Shape the bean mixture into patties using 1-2 heaped table spoons of mixture and gently rolling in flour. If you find the bean mixture to be too mushy, you can add some bread crumbs or a little flour.
- Add a little more oil to the pan and fry the patties over a medium heat, you can fry 2-3 patties at once, cook them for approximately 2 minutes on each side
- Toast and butter the burger buns
- To serve we put all the burger fillings on the table and the kids make their creations

Black beans make great burgers, they give it a very satisfying taste and texture.

Filling variations: *Sliced and lightly fried mushrooms, fried egg, finely chopped pineapple, sliced cooked/tinned beetroot*

SMOOTHIES AND JUICES

Creamy Strawberry Delight

2 cups of fresh spinach
1 cup coconut milk
1 cup coconut water
3 cups strawberries
1 tbsp ground flax seed
1 tsp vanilla extract

- Blend spinach and liquid until smooth.
- Add remaining ingredients, and blend until smooth.

Sweet, Green Monster

Ingredients
2 cups kale
2 cups coconut water
3 cups pineapple
1 cup fresh mint leaves
Juice of 1 lime

- Blend kale and coconut water until smooth.
- Add remaining ingredients, and blend until smooth. Enjoy!

Berry'tastic

2 cups of fresh spinach
1 cup water
1 cup strawberries
1 cup blueberries
1 cup raspberries
2 bananas

- Blend spinach and water until smooth
- Add the remaining fruits and blend again.

Tangy & Velvety Ice Lollies

1 ½ cup fresh spinach
½ cup fresh mint, chopped
¼ cup coconut milk
8 oz frozen bag of strawberries, defrosted
8 oz frozen bag of blueberries, defrosted
¼ cup date syrup

- Blend spinach, mint and coconut milk until smooth
- Add the remaining fruits and blend again
- Pour smoothie into popsicle molds and freeze

Our Special Energizing Green Juice

Makes 2 servings, ***Prep:*** *10 minutes*

50g Kale
4 sticks of celery
1 apple de-cored
½ a cucumber
100g Broccoli
Juicer required

- Wash all vegetables thoroughly
- Peel apple and cucumber
- Juice all items, get energized!

SNACKS

Along with the three main meals, we all need to have snacks in-between meals to help keep our blood sugar stable. This snack would be mid-morning and mid-afternoon. It is best to offer fruit with nuts, veggie sticks with hummus, or even cheese with some oat cakes. When your child is at school, and they have a no nut rule, you can send in seeds instead. The main point is to include some protein with the snack.

Veggie Chips

Makes 5 servings, ***Prep****: 10 minutes,* ***Cooking****: 30 minutes*

500g parsnips

500g sweet potatoes

500g beetroot

Extra light Olive oil

Sea salt and ground black pepper to taste

- Preheat oven to 350 degrees.
- Wash vegetables well
- Slice vegetables very thin, on a slight diagonal and place in a mixing bowl.
- Drizzle lightly with olive oil, salt and pepper and toss so each piece is coated.
- Spread evenly over two baking sheets and place in the oven.
- Remove after 30 minutes or until desired crispness.

Carrot and Zucchini Muffins

Makes 6-9 muffins, ***Prep:*** *15 minutes,* ***Cooking:*** *20 minutes*

1 large carrot, peeled and grated

1 large zucchini, peeled and grated

150g plain flour

2 tsp baking powder

30g light brown sugar

2 egg

¼ cup milk

2 tbsp extra light olive oil

12 hole muffin/cupcake pan

- Preheat the oven to 400F
- Whisk the egg and milk in a bowl
- Mix oil, carrot and zucchini to the milk mixture
- In another bowl shift together the flour and baking powder, then add the sugar
- Combine the two bowls, mixing well
- Line the muffin tray with cases
- Spoon the mixture into each case, filling to about two-thirds
- Bake in the oven for 12 – 15 mins until light brown and firm to touch

Delicious Stovetop Savory Popcorn

In spite of its unappealing name Nutritional Yeast is low in fat and packed with nutrients (particularly B vitamins, folic acid, zinc and protein). Also, as vitamin B12 is not naturally found in plant foods it is a great addition to a vegan diet.

Makes 2 servings, ***Prep:*** *5 minutes,* ***Cooking:*** *5 minutes*

1 tablespoon coconut oil

1/4 cup popcorn kernels

1 tablespoon nutritional yeast

1 tablespoon tamari (gluten free soy sauce)

- Heat oil in a deep, wide sauté pan that you have a lit for.
- Add popcorn and cover.
- Hold pot and shake every few seconds until kernels have popped.
- Remove lid, add tamari and nutritional yeast, mix and transfer to serving bowl.

Energy Balls

These little balls of energy make a great snack for the kids, they are also gluten and dairy free.

1 cup dates

½ cup pumpkin seeds

½ cup sunflower seeds

2 tablespoon vanilla protein powder

1 tablespoon chia seeds

1 tablespoon desiccated coconut flakes

1 teaspoon coconut oil

A pinch of cayenne pepper

¼ cup water

- Mix all the ingredients in a food processor until a dough forms
- Take out a teaspoon of mixture and roll it in your hand
- You can also roll these in other ingredients to enhance the color and flavor, like green tea powder, or desiccated coconut flakes, or cinnamon.
- Store energy balls in the refrigerator for up to two weeks

PART V
BRINGING IT ALL TOGETHER

NUTRITION

I have covered a lot in this book. It may feel overwhelming but any change, however small, is positive. Personally, we eat healthy most of the time, but if the children have a take-out meal, or something sweet now and again, I am not going to panic. I know that they are getting the right nutrients at home, so if they are at a party, I believe they should be allowed to experience it without any restrictions!

1. When you are making the change, you need to schedule it in your diary and make a plan. Only you know how good, or bad your children's diet is, so each step may be different to your own individual family.

2. Look at your child, and see what you need to concentrate on. *Are they overweight, overactive, emotional, tired, sick all the time*? Each child is different, and each person has a tolerance level of what is acceptable and not.

3. You will next write down what a typical 3-day diet looks like, and write it down in a food diary (to download on please visit my website: *www.essentialharmony.net*).

   Is there any area that you can improve on, maybe adding healthy snacks to help stabilize blood sugar, or maybe your child has been missing breakfast? By writing it all down in a diary, will give you an idea on where changes can be made.

4. Map out these changes and when you will implement them. Maybe you will concentrate on one change at a time. Or, all together. You will be the best person to decide this.

5. Once you have decided when the change is going to happen, you need to stick to it, and if your children are old enough, explain to them when and why this is going to happen. Put it in the diary and go for it!

6. Go through all the cupboards, pantry, fridge, freezer and remove any foods that have any ingredients that you cannot pronounce, or if it contains lines, and lines of ingredients. Remove anything with high fructose corn syrup, and anything with trans fats or hydrogenated oils.

7. Plan some meals for the week, including snacks, and that way you know ahead of time what you will be eating. Remember all that you have learned, and be mindful to include as many nutritional foods in the day. This is something I do every Sunday. I plan the whole

week's meals, and then base the food shopping around the list. This was a game changer for our family, as I did not buy anything unnecessarily, nothing ended up going bad, and the food bill dropped too!

8. Children learn by what they see. If you are drinking soda or eating chocolates all day, they will want to as well. This change is a group effort, so please make the change too.

9. It will be hard, but be positive that the changes will benefit your children. As children are adaptable, they will be eating healthier in no time at all.

SOULFUL DIARY, YOGA AND MEDITATION

Including these in your child's daily life will benefit not only the children, but the family as a whole. It will take time to implement them, but please keep at it. You can practice yoga as a family. Children love it when they can do a tree pose for longer than their parents.

1. Print out the diary for the week, so it's ready for the children to fill in (check my website *www.essentialharmony.net* to download one).
2. Make sure they do it every morning and evening; if they find that they can't write, then do it verbally.
3. Encourage them, and fully engage with them when they are filling the diary out. With older children, you can leave them to do it on their own, but keep positive and they will soon love it!
4. With yoga, set a time that you will practice it daily. Communicate with the children so everyone knows that it's yoga time.
5. Let them choose 2-3 poses, and then increase them as and when your children want to. Let them lead it.

6. If it gets out of hand and they cannot focus, then stop and revisit it another day. Remember, it is supposed to be calming.
7. With meditation, get the children to lie down (make sure there is space between the children, to avoid any playful distractions).
8. I would start with reading the meditations, and then try the breathing ones.
9. Every child I know that has tried all three poses have loved it. Please keep at it.

Good Luck! You have taken the first step by reading this book. Now, you are equipped with knowledge that will help you make the necessary changes. Remember, our children are our future.

ABOUT THE AUTHOR

Nishma is a Health Coach, based in Houston, Texas. Her area of expertise is children's health and mother's well-being. She believes that the next generation of children are our future, and we need to ensure that they are nourished not only in their bodies, but their mind and soul as well. She also realizes that motherhood can be difficult, and in some cases, mothers tend to lose their identity.

Steve Jobs once said, "*You can't connect the dots looking forward; you can only connect them looking back.*"

This is how Nishma felt when she looked back through her life. Nishma was a business major, and went on to work at top corporate investment banks. Work was demanding, and after some time, she realized that there was more to life than working all day and most nights with limited energy to do anything else.

When Nishma was in her 20's, she was fortunate to be introduced to the world of yoga, the healing power of reiki (pronounced "RAY-kee") and reflexology. She went on to learn reiki and reflexology, and most of her family and friends thought she was crazy. Why would she add more to her plate, after working so many hours. They questioned why she did this, and Nishma questioned it, too. She had a lucrative paying job that most people would only dream of, and there she was spending all of her spare time learning reiki and reflexology.

Near the end of her banking career, Nishma was actually working both jobs. She would come home from work, and rush to the gym where she was a therapist. It was crazy, but something inside kept her going. Then, one day, Nishma turned in her resignation from the bank. She was getting more pleasure out of helping people heal.

So, there must have been a reason for this craziness. During her time off work, she spent every day for a couple of months visiting her sick grandmother in the hospital. Nishma was grateful for this precious time. She believes that we spend way too much time rushing around that we forget to stop and actually live and spend time with our loved ones.

Not only did Nishma see her gran every day, she also had time to visit with her parents more often. Her gran passed away, and two weeks later, her dad passed away. It was a tough time for the family, but Nishma was thankful for the day she had the courage to resign. It gave her the time she needed to spend with her dear gran and father before they were taken from the family.

She continued working with reflexology and reiki. Reiki is not a cure but it helps shift energy. The vibrations can be strong enough to help change at a cellular level. The treatment is very relaxing, and Nishma's clients come out feeling calm and energized, however, this does not change the underlying health issues. With reflexology, the concept behind it is that every part of your body is represented by a point on your foot. For example, the big toe represents the head. As you press along the foot it, activates the same part in the body. Reflexology is very powerful, especially in children.

Nishma was witnessing far too many adults coming in with one health issue after another. She began to realize that something had to be done to help these clients further. She didn't know then what she knows now—that diet and nutrition is key to optimal well-being.

For Nishma's son, who had a liver transplant when he was a mere 9-months-old, she would practice reiki on him daily to help him heal. He was on immune suppressants to stop his body from rejecting his liver. This drug would unfortunately affect his kidneys. One day, Nishma was massaging her son's feet and she noticed that the 'kidney' point on his feet was red. He was very irritable that day, and she knew something was not right. A visit to the hospital and a lab test later showed that his kidney marker was higher than normal.

So as Steve Job said in relation to the joining the dots of our life together led Nishma to help and heal her son. Even now, both her children love it when she practices reiki or reflexology on them.

Nishma went on to study nutrition in the United Kingdom, and most recently in the United States. During the last nine years, she has focused on making better choices on what she feeds her children. She believes that what we eat leads us to what we become. Providing wholesome nutritious meals gives her children the right nutrients to grown healthy and strong.

Besides focusing on nutrition, Nishma introduced her children to the concept of inner guidance. We all have inner strength and wisdom to lean on in times of uncertainty. Some people resort to food to help them get through stresses but Nishma wanted to teach her children from a young age that through daily journaling and meditation, they can look within for the answers. Finally, through yoga and daily gratitude, she equipped her children with tools that will help them stay emotionally strong.

Nishma has years of experience that she passes on to help both children and mothers. For private coaching, you can find her online at: *www.essentialharmony.net.*

REFERENCES

Chapter 1. Carbohydrates

1. Loren Cordain, et al; *Origins and evolution of the Western diet: health implications for the 21st century*, 2005 February
http://ajcn.nutrition.org/content/81/2/341.long

2. USDA; *Profiling Food Consumption in America*
http://www.usda.gov/factbook/chapter2.pdf

3. The Endocrine Society; *Fructose sugar makes maturing human fat cells fatter, less insulin-sensitive*, 2010 June
http://www.eurekalert.org/pub_releases/2010-06/tes-fsm062010.php

4. Alexandra Shapiro, et al; *Fructose-induced leptin resistance exacerbates weight gain in response to subsequent high-fat feeding*, 2008 November
http://ajpregu.physiology.org/content/295/5/R1370

5. Xiaosen Ouyang, et al; *Fructose consumption as a risk factor for non-alcoholic fatty liver disease*, 2008 June
http://www.journal-of-hepatology.eu/article/S0168-8278(08)00164-5/abstract

6. Bergheim I; *Antibiotics protect against fructose-induced hepatic lipid accumulation in mice: role of endotoxin*, 2008 June
http://www.ncbi.nlm.nih.gov/pubmed/18395289?dopt=Abstract

7. Iozzo P, et al; *Brain PET Imaging in Obesity and Food Addiction: Current Evidence and Hypothesis*, 2012 April
http://www.karger.com/Article/FullText/338328

Chapter 2. Protein

1. Y Wang, MA Beydoun; *Meat consumption is associated with obesity and central obesity among US adults*, 2010 June
http://www.ncbi.nlm.nih.gov/pmc/articles/PMC2697260/

2. Pan A, Sun Q, Bernstein AM, Schulze MB, Manson JE, Stampfer MJ, Willett WC, Hu FB; *Red meat consumption and mortality: results from 2 prospective cohort studies*, 2012 April
www.ncbi.nlm.nih.gov/pubmed/22412075

3. Wilcox S, Sharpe PA, Turner-McGrievy G, Granner M, Baruth M; *Frequency of consumption at fast-food restaurants is associated with dietary intake in overweight and obese women recruited from financially disadvantaged neighborhoods*, 2013 August
www.ncbi.nlm.nih.gov/pubmed/23890353

Chapter 3. Vitamins & Minerals

1. A.D.A.M. Medical Encyclopedia; *Vitamin A*, 2013 February
   www.ncbi.nlm.nih.gov/pubmedhealth/PMH0003052/
2. A.D.A.M. Medical Encyclopedia; *Thiamin*, 2013 February
   www.ncbi.nlm.nih.gov/pubmedhealth/PMH0003053/
3. A.D.A.M. Medical Encyclopedia; *Riboflavin*, 2013 February
   www.ncbi.nlm.nih.gov/pubmedhealth/PMH0003063/
4. A.D.A.M. Medical Encyclopedia; *Niacin*, 2013 February
   www.ncbi.nlm.nih.gov/pubmedhealth/PMH0003061/
5. A.D.A.M. Medical Encyclopedia; *Vitamin B6*, 2013 February
   www.ncbi.nlm.nih.gov/pubmedhealth/PMH0003054/
6. A.D.A.M. Medical Encyclopedia; *Vitamin B12*, 2013 February
   www.ncbi.nlm.nih.gov/pubmedhealth/PMH0003055/
7. Allen LH; *Causes of vitamin B12 and folate deficiency*, 2008 June
   www.ncbi.nlm.nih.gov/pubmed/18709879
8. A.D.A.M. Medical Encyclopedia; *Vitamin C*, 2013 February
   www.ncbi.nlm.nih.gov/pubmedhealth/PMH0003056/
9. A.D.A.M. Medical Encyclopedia; Vitamin D, 2013 February
   www.ncbi.nlm.nih.gov/pubmedhealth/PMH0003057/
10. A.D.A.M. Medical Encyclopedia; , 2013 February
    www.ncbi.nlm.nih.gov/pubmedhealth/PMH0003057/
11. Bikle DD, *Vitamin D and the immune system: role in protection against bacterial infection*, 2008 July
    www.ncbi.nlm.nih.gov/pubmed/18660668

12. A.D.A.M. Medical Encyclopedia; *Vitamin E*, 2013 February
www.ncbi.nlm.nih.gov/pubmedhealth/PMH0003058/

13. A.D.A.M. Medical Encyclopedia; *Vitamin K*, 2013 February
www.ncbi.nlm.nih.gov/pubmedhealth/PMH0003059/

14. More J; *Children's bone health and meeting calcium needs.*, 2008
http://www.ncbi.nlm.nih.gov/pubmed/18494428

15. Miller GD; *The importance of meeting calcium needs with foods*, 2001 April
http://www.ncbi.nlm.nih.gov/pubmed/11349940

16. Walter Mertz; *Chromium in Human Nutriton*, 2014 December
http://jn.nutrition.org/content/123/4/626.long

17. A.D.A.M. Medical Encyclopedia; Anemia caused by low iron – children, 2014 February
http://www.ncbi.nlm.nih.gov/pubmedhealth/PMH0004451/

18. A.D.A.M. Medical Encyclopedia;Influence of selenium on innate immune response in kids
http://www.ncbi.nlm.nih.gov/pubmed/20140724

19. S Maggini Essential Role of Vitamin C and Zinc in Child Immunity and Health
http://imr.sagepub.com/content/38/2/386.long

Chapter 4. Fats

1. Simopoulos AP; *The importance of the ratio of omega-6/omega-3 essential fatty acids*, 2002 October
   www.ncbi.nlm.nih.gov/pubmed/12442909

2. Kaitosaari T1, et al; *Low-saturated fat dietary counseling starting in infancy improves insulin sensitivity in 9-year-old healthy children: the Special Turku Coronary Risk Factor Intervention Project for Children (STRIP) study*, 2006 April
   www.ncbi.nlm.nih.gov/pubmed/16567815

3. Ryan T. Hurt, MD, PhD, et al; *The Obesity Epidemic: Challenges, Health Initiatives, and Implications for Gastroenterologists*, 2010 Dec
   www.ncbi.nlm.nih.gov/pmc/articles/PMC3033553/

4. V Marchand; *Trans fats: What physicians should know*, 2010 July
   www.ncbi.nlm.nih.gov/pmc/articles/PMC2921725/

5. Food and Drug Administration; *Guidance for Industry: Trans Fatty Acids in Nutrition Labeling, Nutrient Content Claims, Health Claims; Small Entity Compliance Guide*, 2003 August
   www.fda.gov/Food/GuidanceRegulation/GuidanceDocumentsRegulatoryInformation/LabelingNutrition/ucm053479.htm

Chapter 5. Drinks

1. USGS; *The water in you*, 2014 March
   http://water.usgs.gov/edu/propertyyou.html
2. Barry M. Popkin, et al; *Water, Hydration and Health*, 2011 August
   www.ncbi.nlm.nih.gov/pmc/articles/PMC2908954/
3. Lars Järup; *Hazards of heavy metal contamination*, 2003
   http://bmb.oxfordjournals.org/content/68/1/167.long
4. Rehydration after Exercise with Fresh young Coconut Water,
   www.jstage.jst.go.jp/article/jpa/21/2/21_2_93/_pdf
5. Babey SH, et al; *Bubbling over: soda consumption and its link to obesity in California* 2009 September
   www.ncbi.nlm.nih.gov/pubmed/19768858
6. Hippokratia; *Is beverage intake related to overweight and obesity in school children?*
   www.ncbi.nlm.nih.gov/pmc/articles/PMC3738277/pdf/hippokratia-17-42.pdf
7. Marcella L, et al; *Soda Consumption and Overweight Status of 2-Year-Old Mexican-American Children in California*, 2006 November
   www.onlinelibrary.wiley.com/doi/10.1038/oby.2006.230/full
8. Nicklas TA; *Eating patterns, dietary quality and obesity*, 2001 Dec
   http://www.ncbi.nlm.nih.gov/pubmed/11771675

Chapter 6. The Digestive System

1. G Vighi, et al; *Allergy and the gastrointestinal system*, 2008 September www.ncbi.nlm.nih.gov/pmc/articles/PMC2515351/
2. Dinesh S. Pashankar; *Childhood Constipation: Evaluation and Management*, 2005 May www.ncbi.nlm.nih.gov/pmc/articles/PMC2780136/
3. Kirsi M. Järvinen, et al; *Intestinal permeability in children with food allergy on specific elimination diets* 2013 August http://onlinelibrary.wiley.com/enhanced/doi/10.1111/pai.12106/
4. Melissa Lee Phillips; *Gut Reaction: Environmental Effects on the Human Microbiota*, 2009 May www.ncbi.nlm.nih.gov/pmc/articles/PMC2685866/
5. Josef Neu, Jona Rushing; *Cesarean versus Vaginal Delivery: Long term infant outcomes and the Hygiene Hypothesis*, 2011 June www.ncbi.nlm.nih.gov/pmc/articles/PMC3110651/
6. Scott Gilbert; *A holobiont birth narrative: the epigenetic transmission of the human microbiome*, 2014 August www.ncbi.nlm.nih.gov/pmc/articles/PMC4137224/
7. J. Marc Rhoads, et al; *Altered Fecal Microflora and Increased Fecal Calprotectin in Infants with Colic*, 2009 December http://www.jpeds.com/article/S0022-3476(09)00487-9/abstract
8. Thomas Koonce, et al; Colicky baby? *Here's a surprising remedy*, 2011 January http://www.ncbi.nlm.nih.gov/pmc/articles/PMC3183958/
9. Savino F; *Intestinal microflora in breastfed colicky and non-colicky infants*, 2004 June http://www.ncbi.nlm.nih.gov/pubmed/15244234

10. Hill MJ; *Intestinal flora and endogenous vitamin synthesis*, 1997 March http://www.ncbi.nlm.nih.gov/pubmed/9167138

11. Michele M. KosiewiczGut; *Microbiota, Immunity, and Disease: A Complex Relationship*, 2011 September http://www.ncbi.nlm.nih.gov/pmc/articles/PMC3166766/

12. Sherwood L. Gorbach; *Microbiology of the Gastrointestinal Tract*, 1996 http://www.ncbi.nlm.nih.gov/books/NBK7670/

Chapter 7. Brain

1. Fernando Gómez-Pinilla; *Brain foods: the effects of nutrients on brain function*, 2010 January www.ncbi.nlm.nih.gov/pmc/articles/PMC2805706/
2. Rada P, Avena NM, Hoebel BG; *Daily bingeing on sugar repeatedly releases dopamine in the accumbens shell*, 2005 www.ncbi.nlm.nih.gov/pubmed/15987666
3. Chang CY, Ke DS, Chen JY; *Essential fatty acids and human brain,* 2009 December www.ncbi.nlm.nih.gov/pubmed/20329590
4. Simon N. Young; *How to increase serotonin in the human brain without drugs*, 2007 December www.ncbi.nlm.nih.gov/pmc/articles/PMC2077351/
5. Fernstrom JD; *Effects on the diet on brain neurotransmitters*, 1977 February www.ncbi.nlm.nih.gov/pubmed/13261
6. Medin T, Rinholm JE, Owe SG, Sagvolden T, Gjedde A, Storm-Mathisen J, Bergersen LH; *Low dopamine D5 receptor density in hippocampus in an animal model of attention-deficit/hyperactivity disorder (ADHD)*, 2013 July www.ncbi.nlm.nih.gov/pubmed/23541742
7. Jason Yanofski; *The Dopamine Dilemma*, 2010 June www.ncbi.nlm.nih.gov/pmc/articles/PMC2898838/
8. Michael Camilleri; *Serotonin in the Gastrointestinal Tract*, 2010 February http://www.ncbi.nlm.nih.gov/pmc/articles/PMC2694720/
9. Kaplan BJ, et al; *Vitamins, minerals, and mood*, 2007 September http://ncbi.nlm.nih.gov/pubmed/17723028

Chapter 8. Immune

1. G Vighi, et al; *Allergy and the gastrointestinal system*, 2008 September
www.ncbi.nlm.nih.gov/pmc/articles/PMC2515351/
2. Purchiaroni F, et al; *The role of intestinal microbiota and the immune system*, 2013 February
www.ncbi.nlm.nih.gov/pubmed/23426535
3. Fasano A, Shea-Donohue T; *Mechanisms of disease: the role of intestinal barrier function in the pathogenesis of gastrointestinal autoimmune diseases*, 2005 September
www.ncbi.nlm.nih.gov/pubmed/16265432
4. Odenwald MA, Turner JR; *Intestinal permeability defects: is it time to treat?* 2013 September
www.ncbi.nlm.nih.gov/pubmed/23851019
5. Fatemeh Rafii, et al; *Effects of treatment with antimicrobial agents on the human colonic microflora* 2008 December
www.ncbi.nlm.nih.gov/pmc/articles/PMC2643114/
6. Calder PC, Kew S; *The immune system: a target for functional foods?* 2002 November
www.ncbi.nlm.nih.gov/pubmed/12495459

CPSIA information can be obtained
at www.ICGtesting.com
Printed in the USA
LVOW04s1313270716
497997LV00025B/550/P